Guy Jobin
Spirituality in the Biomedical World

Studies in Spiritual Care

Edited by
Simon Peng-Keller, Eckhard Frick,
Christina Puchalski, and John Swinton

Volume 5

Guy Jobin

Spirituality in the Biomedical World

Moving between Order and "Subversion"

DE GRUYTER

ISBN 978-3-11-052526-7
e-ISBN (PDF) 978-3-11-063895-0
e-ISBN (EPUB) 978-3-11-063920-9
ISSN 2511-8838

Library of Congress Control Number: 2020935258

Bibliographic information published by the Deutsche Nationalbibliothek
The Deutsche Nationalbibliothek lists this publication in the Deutsche Nationalbibliografie;
detailed bibliographic data are available in the Internet at http://dnb.dnb.de.

© 2020 Walter de Gruyter GmbH, Berlin/Boston
Printing: CPI books GmbH, Leck

www.degruyter.com

Table of Contents

Part II. The "subversive" nature of spirituality in healthcare

List of Tables

https://doi.org/10.1515/9783110638950-001

1 Introduction

Why talk about spirituality in connection with the world of healthcare? The question will seem pointless to some, and self-evident to others. First, of course, it will seem pointless to anyone inside or outside healthcare who looks at only the technical and scientific aspects. Why include spirituality, a fuzzy, hard-to-define and unquantifiable notion, as a focus of healthcare? From this point of view, spirituality has no connection with biomedical science and the care options it provides. Second, the same question will seem self-evident to anyone who considers healthcare to be a holistic action which, like illness itself, affects the whole person and not just the body. For this group, it is obvious that healthcare must take into account, and even put to use, the sick person's spiritual experience.

Both attitudes can be experienced in the healthcare world, at least in Western countries. The degree to which one takes precedence over the other varies, from one care sector and one institution to another. However, in institutions open to the spiritual experience, spirituality is increasingly considered as something that must be taken into account by caregivers, obviously within the boundaries of their own professional discipline. And, going beyond the level of personal initiatives, the need for healthcare teams as a whole to pay attention to what patients experience at the spiritual level has been increasingly recognized in recent years.[1]

The need to take the spiritual experience during illness into account is part of a broader trend in Western societies—a fascination with the practical uses of spirituality and its contribution to individual wellbeing, whether through a religious or a humanist tradition. As portrayed in the mass media and specialized literature aimed at the general public,[2] the contemporary interest in spirituality appears to have replaced religion as the main vector for meaning in Western societies that have "departed from religion", to paraphrase philosopher Marcel Gauchet.[3] From these clues, it is possible to deduce that the spiritual question

---

1 Christina M. Puchalski et al., "Interdisciplinary spiritual care for seriously ill and dying patients: a collaborative model," *Cancer J* 12, no. 5 (2006); Christina M. Puchalski and Betty Ferrell, *Making Health Care Whole. Integrating Spirituality into Patient Care* (West Conshohocken, Pa: Templeton Press, 2010).
2 This explosion in spiritual literature is part of the creation of a lucrative market in spirituality-related books, magazines, websites, support groups, etc.
3 Marcel Gauchet, *Le désenchantement du monde: une histoire politique de la religion* (Paris: Gallimard, 1985). I say "appears" because sociological studies of spirituality show that although it is clearly present in contemporary culture, this does not necessarily mean that "spiritual" people

https://doi.org/10.1515/9783110638950-002

is increasingly a component in the institutional structures and cultural representations of Western societies. I will use the term "spiritual question" in this book to refer to all aspects of the attention paid, in the healthcare world, to the spiritual experience during illness. Included as components of the "spiritual question" are: the intellectual exercise of defining spirituality and theorizing its connection with existing religious traditions; the problems caused by the drive to institutionalize consideration for the spiritual experience during a period of illness, and the attempts made by organizations to solve those problems; the development of knowledge and clinical tools to take the spiritual experience into account during a period of illness; the drafting of legislative and regulatory instruments to provide a framework for spiritual and religious support in care settings; and so on. Like social issues in the 19th century, and sexual issues in the 20th and 21st centuries, the spiritual question has emerged in the wake of a social and cultural movement. Last, it is important to note that the spiritual question is not confined to the world of healthcare; it also affects the business management[4] and education[5] sectors.

1.1 Link to contemporary culture

The world of healthcare is closely entwined with contemporary culture, and therefore also affected by the general fascination with the spiritual question, but for its own reasons. First, the link between contemporary culture and healthcare is created by the preponderant role played by healthcare institutions in the

---

outnumber "religious" people, cf. Paul Heelas and Linda Woodhead, *The spiritual revolution: why religion is giving way to spirituality* (Malden, MA: Blackwell Pub, 2005); Jörg Stolz et al., *Religion et spiritualité à l'ère de l'ego: profils de l'institutionnel, de l'alternatif, du distancié et du séculier [Religion and spirituality in the era of the ego. Institutional, alternative, distancing and secular profiles]* (Genève: Labor et Fides, 2015).

4 Thierry C. Pauchant and Le Forum international sur le management l'éthique et la spiritualité, *Pour un management éthique et spirituel: défis, cas, outils et questions* (Saint-Laurent, Québec: Fides, 2000); Thierry C. Pauchant and Le Forum international sur le management l'éthique et la spiritualité, *Ethics and spirituality at work: hopes and pitfalls of the search for meaning in organizations* (Westport, Conn: Quorum Books, 2002); Ian I. Mitroff and Elizabeth A. Denton, *A spiritual audit of corporate America: a hard look at spirituality, religion, and values in the workplace*, 1st ed. (San Francisco: Jossey-Bass Publishers, 1999).

5 Terence Copley, *Spiritual development in the State school: a perspective on worship and spirituality in the education system of England and Wales* (Exeter: University of Exeter Press, 2000); Andrew Wright, *Spirituality and education* (London: Falmer Press, 2000).

emergence of what has been called the therapy society,[6] or, at the very least, the culture of support, of which therapeutic support is a major component.[7] This is the culture in which a person who feels vulnerable in his or her personal, professional or social life can rely on the expertise of an individual or institution for assistance in coping with a physical, mental or, once again, social problem. The role of the therapist is to provide support for vulnerability. This idea can be extended theoretically to suggest that in a therapy society, therapy can be seen as a "total social fact", to borrow an expression from French sociologist Marcel Mauss,[8] in other words as something that fundamentally structures relationships between individuals and between individuals and institutions. In a society that is seen as being aggressive towards individuals by placing too many requirements on them—to the point where A. Ehrenberg has written about the "fatigue of being oneself"[9] and the "unease-inducing society"[10]— healing, or at least support along the path towards some form of healing, becomes an objective and a process of self-reappropriation.

1.2 A health-based logic

However, the idea that we live in a therapy-based culture is not the only reason for addressing the spiritual question in healthcare institutions, since the conditions in which care is provided also provide an incentive to address the issue. Without giving an exhaustive list, the conditions include those given below, which will be investigated at more length in later sections of the book. They are expressed in the form of paradoxes.

First, the very nature of healthcare institutions plays a role. Spirituality is a welcome addition to a highly technical and highly bureaucratic world that is, nevertheless, dedicated to the healing of flesh-and-bones individuals. The con-

---

6 Philip Rieff, *The Triumph of the Therapeutic. Uses of Faith after Freud* (Chicago: University of Chicago Press, 1966); Joel J. Shuman and Keith G. Meador, *Heal Thyself. Spirituality, Medicine, and the Distorsion of Christianity* (Oxford: Oxford University Press, 2003); Jonathan B. Imber, ed. *Therapeutic Culture. Triumph and Defeat* (Herndon, VA: Transaction, 2004).

7 Tanguy Châtel, "Les nouvelles cultures de l'accompagnement: les soins palliatifs, une voie 'spirituelle' dans une société de performance" (École Pratique des Hautes Études, 2008), tome 1, 203–23.

8 Marcel Mauss, "Essai sur le don. Forme et raison de l'échange dans les sociétés archaïques," in *Sociologie et anthropologie*, ed. Marcel Mauss (Paris: Quadrige/Presses universitaires de France, 2004[1950]): 274–76.

9 Alain Ehrenberg, *La fatigue d'être soi: dépression et société* (Paris: O. Jacob, 1998).

10 Alain Ehrenberg, *La société du malaise* (Paris: Odile Jacob, 2010).

trast, and even the antinomy, between caring for a suffering body, unique in every case, and the cold technical environment in which care is provided, is one of the anchor points for the spiritual question in healthcare institutions. Whatever the institution has lost in "humanity" will, according to this approach, be compensated for and even reinstated by an ongoing focus on a patient's spiritual experience, and by the attention paid by the institution to the spiritual experience of its caregivers. After all, the spiritual dimension can be one of the many inputs in the choice of a profession and in professional identity.[11]

Secondly, the biomedical world relies on evidence-based medicine and a scientific approach. Science, like other modern-day disciplines, has made its own contribution to the disenchantment of the world,[12] in other words the loss of credibility of religious or magical explanations of the physical and human world.[13] On the other hand, the biomedical world has, in several care sectors and thanks to palliative care, discovered or rediscovered the holistic reality of each sick person. There is now recognition for the fact that the effects of illness have impacts on the person's body, mind and social and family relationships.[14] These dimensions of human life have become part of the focus of care; in other words, they receive professional attention from caregivers.

Third, healthcare institutions in many Western societies were originally founded by religious or philanthropic groups. In both cases, the value systems of the founding group left a mark on the institutional culture and the focus of care. At the same time, these value systems determined the nature of the medical approaches that could be practised. It is possible to state that the monotheist traditions (Judaism, Christianity, Islam) continued to support institutional caregiving in the West and in some societies, including Québec, until the mid-20th century. In addition to this support, it is important to note that in the institutions founded by religious groups, the relevant religious rites for times of illness or imminent death were provided alongside medical care.

---

11 Charles G. Sasser and Christina M. Puchalski, "The humanistic clinician: traversing the science and art of health care," *J Pain Symptom Manage* 39, no. 5 (2010); Daniel P. Sulmasy, *The Healer's Calling. A Spirituality for Physicians and Other Health Care Professionals* (Mahwah, N.J.: Paulist Press, 1997).

12 Ilya Prigogine and Isabelle Stengers, *La nouvelle alliance: métamorphose de la science* (Paris: Gallimard, 1980).

13 Gauchet, *Le désenchantement du monde: une histoire politique de la religion*; Max Weber, *L'éthique protestante et l'esprit du capitalisme* (Paris: Plon, 1964).

14 George L. Engel, "The need for a new medical model: a challenge for biomedicine," *Science* 196, no. 4286 (1977).

In the 20th century, the situation began to change, leading to a shift in the relationship between religion and healthcare institutions. The secularization of Western culture was often reflected in organizational structures by the laicization of the governance and day-to-day operations of the institutions making up "the basic structure of society—the main political and social institutions and the way they fit together as one scheme of cooperation."[15] Healthcare institutions form part of this basic structure, even more so when the societies they serve are imbued with a therapy culture.

The two influences outlined above, one from the prevailing culture and one from the world of healthcare, combine and make it possible to include the spiritual question in the actual organization of Western healthcare institutions. The institutions pledge to include in their organizational structure a focus on the impacts of illness and medical care on the patient's spiritual experience; a focus, of one kind or another, on the patient's "spiritual resources" in the care plan;[16] and recognition of the patient's, and the patient's family's, need to experience illness in a way that goes beyond a strictly physiological or psychological approach. Quebec offers a clear example of this institutional openness, since one of the fundamental pieces of legislation that deals with the organization and delivery of care in healthcare institutions requires them to take their patients' spiritual needs into account.[17]

1.3 Spirituality, public use of reason, secularization

It may appear surprising that institutions are responsible for this interest in spirituality, especially in a culture in which spiritual matters are generally seen as a

---

15 John Rawls, *La justice comme équité. Une reformulation de Théorie de la justice* (Montréal: Boréal, 2004), 21.

16 This may extend to changing an initial or habitual care plan to take into account, as far as possible, the patient's religious and spiritual beliefs and any related imperatives.

17 "The function of institutions is to ensure the provision of safe, continuous and accessible quality health or social services which respect the rights and spiritual needs of individuals and which aim at reducing or solving health and welfare problems and responding to the needs of the various population groups. To that end, institutions must manage their human, material, information, technological and financial resources effectively and efficiently and cooperate with other key players, including community organizations, to act on health and social determinants and improve the supply of services to the public. In addition, a local authority must elicit and facilitate such cooperation." "S-4.2 Loi sur les services de santé et les services sociaux," ed. Ministère de la santé et des services sociaux (Québec: Gouvernement du Québec, 2005), section 100.

strictly individual concern. In fact, sociologically speaking the difference between a religious culture and a "spiritual" culture is what Heelas and Woodhead have called the subjective turn.[18] This cultural shift is, in their view, "a turn away from life lived in terms of external or 'objective' roles, duties and obligations, and a turn towards life lived by reference to one's own subjective experience."[19] One's own "self" is no longer seen as the place where an ideal life defined by tradition and imposed from the outside is updated, but rather as the very source of the ideal life. This description follows on from the sociological tradition inaugurated by Thomas Luckmann, for whom the individualization of belief was the marker for the transformation from religious life to modernity.[20] The fact that religion has been made invisible in the modern lifestyle coincides with its relegation to the private sphere, outside the bounds of the public sphere. The healthcare world's interest in spirituality calls this interpretation into question, since it shows that spirituality, instead of being relegated to the private sphere, has now acquired a public dimension—and, in addition, in laicized institutions.

1.4 Place in institutions

The "arrival" of the spiritual question in the healthcare world has been welcomed by a large majority of stakeholders and observers of healthcare trends. This enthusiasm extends to the fields of both clinical care and research. As we will see in later chapters, various reasons are given for the support shown by caregivers for the inclusion of spirituality in the range of care provided. However, the main reason is clearly the fact that they perceive and interpret it as having beneficial effects for both sides of the care relationship (patient/caregiver), for the care relationship itself, and for the institution. Enthusiasm in the research field is reflected in the growing number of studies and publications that analyze and determine the conditions, mechanisms and effects of integrating spirituality into healthcare. A close reading of the biomedical literature on the spiritual question quickly reveals a major focus—to extend and integrate the inclusion of spirituality in order to improve the care provided. However, it is important to note the small number of critical studies in this research area. With few exceptions, the research that has been published is always in some way favourable to even more integration. This will be covered in more detail later. It may be that

---

18 Heelas and Woodhead, *The spiritual revolution: why religion is giving way to spirituality*, 2–5.
19 Heelas and Woodhead, *The spiritual revolution: why religion is giving way to spirituality*, 2.
20 Thomas Luckmann, *The Invisible Religion. The Problem of Religion in Modern Society* (New York: MacMillan, 1967).

this situation is typical of an emerging field of research and reflects the fact that the institutionalization of the spiritual question is still at a crucial phase where the most effort is directed at gaining recognition for the field in an institutional sector still offering some resistance, as I mentioned above. Research therefore tends to emphasize the relevance of integrating spirituality for institutions, and also demonstrate the clinical advantages it brings.

1.5 Questions

Despite the clear strong fascination with the inclusion of spirituality in health-care, the approach is still questioned. The questions can be sociological, anthro-pological, political, epistemological or theological in nature, and it is worth cit-ing some of them here, in the same order. What does the inclusion of spirituality say about the Western relationship with religion and the question of meaning? What representation of human beings underlies the welcome offered by the in-stitutional and clinical sectors of biomedical practice? In a given jurisdiction, what are the links between the type of laicity established and the approach taken to the spiritual question by the healthcare institutions concerned? What exactly does biomedical research include in the "spirituality" category? What is the relationship between the religious and spiritual traditions that have marked the Western world and the "spirituality" construct of biomedical culture?

All of these questions exceed the scope of this book, but should, in my opin-ion, be addressed by a program of critical research on the integration of spiritu-ality in the healthcare world.

1.6 Objectives

This book targets a modest objective, but one that lies within the program of crit-ical research outlined above. Taking a critical standpoint, while remaining aware of the "subversive" potential of spiritual life with respect to any form of institu-tionalization, the goal is to:
1) define the place occupied by spirituality in the healthcare world;
2) describe the role and functions assigned to spirituality by healthcare institu-tions;

3) identify some of the limitations inherent in any attempt to institutionalize something as evanescent and fleeting as spiritual life;[21]
4) discuss some of the categories (care sectors, care professions, care protocols and policies) that govern the institutionalization of the spiritual question in the healthcare world.

These objectives support the general aim of the book, which is to show that the spiritual question and the ways in which it is introduced into healthcare institutions tend to oscillate between the twin poles of order (by helping achieve the mission of the healthcare institution) and disruption (by overstepping the strict limits set by the clinical and research components of biomedical culture).

For this reason, Part One will be devoted to the question of order. It will examine some of the conditions that apply to consideration for, and the introduction of, the spiritual question into the healthcare culture. Part Two will show that, even if a form of integration has been achieved, it does not exhaust the spiritual questions involved and, above all, may ignore the "subversive" potential of spirituality, in other words its potential ability to destabilize organizational approaches that are over-confident and focused on control.

---

21 "Limitations" are inherent in any process of institutionalization. An institution's rules restrict the actions that an individual or community may take in various situations. However, institutionalization is not necessarily "negative" since it ensures consistency over time, or at least stability in the actions that require social cooperation. In this, sociological, meaning of the term, institutionalization is both a brake on and a facilitator for social action.

Part I. **Order, or the sapientialization of the spiritual experience**

2 About wisdom

The spiritual question is introduced into the healthcare world along a very specific path. This path, which involves what I call "the sapientialization of the spiritual experience," requires the spiritual experience, whether individual or collective, to be expressed under the auspices of and in terms of wisdom. Before explaining in more detail what I mean by a wisdom discourse, it is important to note that it is a trait of religious experience that is recognized by religious tradition and theological discourse. Several theologians and many specialists of religious traditions recognize two main types of religious discourse: wisdom discourse and prophetic discourse.

> Wisdom [...] is, first, a reasoned discourse about the cosmos, at least the parts of it accessible to human investigation: astral bodies and worlds, including our own planet; the Earth and its domains—animal, vegetable and mineral; and the human beings that inhabit, cultivate, explore, and benefit from it. At this level, wisdom is science... More profoundly, wisdom concerns itself with what is invisible, what is manifest in each of the Earth's movements but cannot be grasped in itself: force, energy, resistance, the spiritual world—examples include angels and the human soul. Next, wisdom studies human behaviour by observing it, but also by attempting to define its principles of action; wisdom becomes the art of living, and morality. Last, it turns to God and examines the possibility of speaking of Him not only as the cornerstone of all reality, but in His actual divinity, to the extent that we can reach this far and discuss it; it becomes "metaphysical", in other words a language that attempts to describe things that are either absolutely beyond, or totally beneath, our habitual fields of investigation. In this way, wisdom seeks to understand the coherence of each and all levels of being and existence, and to perceive their harmony. Unlike prophecy, it places less emphasis on disconnection than on connection, articulation, harmony or, in a word: order.[1]

According to theologian Ghislain Lafont, wisdom has three modes: a cosmological discourse on the way the world is organized, an ethical discourse on the conduct of human life, and a metaphysical discourse that takes the form of a rational discourse about God. All three share a common trait: the notion of order, that can be identified in the world by reason. The coherence that reason seeks to identify is the foundation that gives meaning to individual and collective human life. In other words, from a wisdom-based perspective, order provides meaning.

---

1 Ghislain Lafont, *La sagesse et la prophétie. Modèles théologiques* (Paris: Cerf, 1999), 18–19.

https://doi.org/10.1515/9783110638950-003

In his analysis of sapiential texts from the Old Testament, US exegete James Crenshaw identifies three ways of understanding meaning, associated with wisdom:[2]

1) A wisdom discourse is characterized by a search for the meaning of life that goes beyond each individual. What Crenshaw calls the natural discourse is the component of wisdom that involves a search for order in the universe, which is at first glance hidden but can be discerned through the application of reasoning. The focus is not necessarily order itself, but its potential for harmonization. By identifying our place in a pre-existing order, we can become part of a network of meaning that gives direction and significance to the events that affect us and the actions that we take. Cosmology provides meaning.

2) The second aspect of meaning is based on ethics. The wisdom discourse presents the wise man as a reference for others, and as someone who has reflected, on the basis of his own life, successes and failures, on what makes a happy human being and a good life. Obviously, the criteria for a good life or happiness vary from one culture to another. One society may place the emphasis on the virtue of courage, while another may propose virtues that are more suited to deliberation and decision-making. For example, biblical wisdom sets out the following features of a good life: longevity, good health, material comfort, a large number of descendants, and a good reputation. In the words of Crenshaw, this is an experiential discourse. I would prefer to describe it as a discourse on happiness and a good life.

In addition, the ideal characteristics of a good life are presented alongside a discourse that questions the meaning of life, often triggered by undeserved suffering (one example is Job and his friends) and the oppressive shadows of death (Kohelet).[3]

3) The third and last theme is a reflection on the injustices of life and the limits on the ability of human reason to discern its meaning, which I refer to as a discourse of theodicy. In the Judeo-Christian tradition, Job is once again the emblematic figure of this form of wisdom. Theodicy is the hallmark of a metaphysical discourse, in the definition given by Lafont.

---

2 James L. Crenshaw, "Wisdom Literature," in *The Oxford Companion to the Bible*, ed. Bruce M. Metzger and Michael D. Coogan (New York: Oxford University Press, 1993): 801–03.
3 Crenshaw, "Wisdom Literature": 802.

It is possible to conclude that, as far as wisdom is concerned, the discourse of systematic theology and the discourse of biblical exegesis mirror one another.

The ethical aspect of wisdom is clearly the most audible in the modern world, characterized by the "disenchantment" produced by science and secularization. In this case, wisdom is seen for its practical possibilities. In his article on "Wisdom" in the *Dictionnaire encyclopédique d'éthique chrétienne*, Jesùs Asurmendy indicates that the idea of wisdom is closely related to the notion of a good life: "Each civilization may have its own form of wisdom, but in all cases it involves achieving a good life, in and by wisdom. [...] Wisdom is knowledge, knowledge about how to do things that leads to [...] knowledge about how to achieve a good life."[4] Wisdom is a form of knowledge that identifies regularity, the "laws" that, in an ordered world, signpost the path towards achievement and a good life. These laws—identified and formulated via the activity of contemplating the real world, what the Ancient Greeks called *theoria*—can be sought both in human nature and in the cosmos, based on the assumption that they possess a form of universality, as long as they are identified by reason, and not by reliance on a specific form of revelation. Once again according to Asurmendy, "it is not surprising that wisdom is closely focused on the cosmos and the created world. Order, organization, and regularity attract the wise man. By understanding them, he is able to identify the rules that govern the world in which he lives and to distill the instructions and prescriptions he will need to achieve a good life."[5]

This means that, for the wise man, theoretical activity will lead to practical action which will, in turn, become an integral part of the contemplated order. The wise man will move from *theoria* to *praxis* in order to integrate into the order of the world of which he already forms a part.

The key point here is that the practice of wisdom targets a dual coherency: first, coherency with oneself by conforming to one's human nature and the "laws" that govern personal growth and, second, coherency with the cosmos and creation, through integration. These are the two aspects of a good life.

A wisdom discourse results from the observation and identification of the indicators for the relationships, organization and coherency between the various elements that make up the world. The discourse embodies, in its own way, an understanding of the world that presupposes an organizing and unifying principle for phenomena that appear, *prima faciae*, to reflect diversity and plurality.

---

4 Jesus Asurmendy, "Sagesse," in *Dictionnaire encyclopédique d'éthique chrétienne*, ed. Laurent Lemoine, Eric Gaziaux, and Denis Müller (Paris: Cerf, 2013): 1795.
5 Asurmendy, "Sagesse": 1801.

The principle has been given several different names in Western history: God, Providence (in both Christian tradition and the preceding Stoic tradition), Nature, the Cosmos, etc.

2.1 The hypothesis of sapientialisation

At first sight, the hypothesis of the sapientialisation of the spiritual experience in the world of biomedicine appears to be an artificial construct. Biomedicine seems to be diametrically opposed to the wisdom discourse. Any parallel between the two forms of knowledge of the surrounding world appears difficult to establish, given the gulf between a form of practical and speculative wisdom, on the one hand, and the biomedical technosciences, on the other. First, the mission of biomedicine is not to produce a metaphysical discourse, like some schools of theology or philosophy.[6] It is a discipline based on experimental and fundamental science with an eminently practical goal: 1) to prevent illness and injury and promote and maintain health; 2) to ease the pain and suffering caused by illness; 3) to care for and cure the sick, and to care for people who cannot be cured; and 4) to prevent premature death and provide for a peaceful death.[7] The biomedical sciences are not a form of ethics. Secondly, biomedicine does not simply comply with the "laws of the real world", and is not content to be simply a detached observer, powerless to intervene in healthy or pathological processes. On the contrary, it ardently wants to intervene and even control bodies and healthy and pathological processes. It clearly intends to change the course of human life, and has been successful in doing so. Thanks to the biomedical research conducted in the early 20th century, deadly illnesses of the time such as tuberculosis, could be cured; malformations, whether innate or acquired, could be corrected by surgery; and so on.

It is true that biomedicine is not wisdom in the classical meaning of the term; its primary mission is not to indicate to individuals and communities how to live a good moral life. However, biomedicine does share a common objective with the wisdom discourse, namely to discover the "laws" that govern the organization of the real world, in this case the laws of the human body and mind. Obviously, biomedicine is not seeking a primal cause or extraneous

---

6 The most obvious example of this type of overarching discourse is the work of the scholastic theologies and philosophies taught at universities in the Middle Ages.

7 "The Goals of Medicine: Setting New Priorities. Special Supplement," *The Hastings Center Report* 26, no. 6 (1996): S1–S27. The article presents the results of an international consensus conference organized by the Hastings Center for Bioethics in 1996.

principle of organization. It limits its scope to the identification of recurrences, relations, and the ordering of causal relationships between observable phenomena. Nevertheless, it still attempts to identify an order in the way in which the human body reacts to illness.

In addition, even though biomedicine takes the stance of an active agent that can "overstep" the "laws of the real world" that appeared until very recently to be insurmountable barriers,[8] it is also a creator of order. As we will see in the next chapter, biomedicine has modified the representations and realities that were until recently beyond the grasp of pre-modern medicine. In this area, medicine re-orders realities such as the representations of life and death, health and sickness, responsibility and chance that structure contemporary thought. In fact, this is a re-ordering, or the creation of a different form of order, but one that remains an order. Biomedicine has put in place a new order, no longer the order of Nature alone, but of an "assisted" Nature, since Nature is now scrutinized in its most detailed aspects.

And it is within this new order that the spiritual experience during illness must be integrated, within this "wisdom" of the body and mind that biomedicine has recreated.

---

8 In particular, when the healing or mitigation of symptoms changes the "natural" course of the illness.

3 A new biomedical order?

Biomedicine occupies an important place in the lives of citizens in Western societies. It has acquired a status and power that are practically equivalent to those enjoyed by the Christian churches prior to the modern era. One tangible sign that biomedicine has taken the place of the churches is the fact that overall health—meaning a person's physical and mental, and also spiritual, health—has become the new figure of salvation.[1] The Christian churches presented salvation—in other words the ultimate accomplishment of a human being—as the survival of the human self after physical death, purified from sin and in the presence of God. However, with the decline of the religious traditions, this "supernatural" representation of salvation has been replaced by a more "earthly" vision of health as the new salvation. As a result, people today strive just as much as their religious forbears to obtain salvation—the difference being that salvation now occurs in the here and now rather than in the hereafter.

This shift from the traditional Christian viewpoint to the current discourse can be seen in two concomitant and interwoven movements. The first is the "grounding of salvation", the idea that salvation now literally occurs on Earth. In sociology, this would be referred to as "intramondanisation." Salvation, today, occurs in strictly human terms of health, as defined by the biomedical world. The second movement involves seeing health not as an analogy of salvation, as it is in the Gospels, but as being equivalent to salvation, as it is in the contemporary discourse. In the evangelical approach health is, *due proportion being observed*, an image of future salvation, but physical health, as experienced during a human lifetime, is incommensurate with salvation itself. This analogical discourse is based on *could be*, emphasizing a link between the two objects of comparison but, at the same time, their radical dissimilarity. The contemporary discourse on wellbeing, in the so-called therapy society,[2] relies not on *could be* but on *is*. Health *is* salvation—the two elements in the equation are bal-

---

1 "Health replaces salvation, said Guardia. This is because medicine offers modern man the obstinate, yet reassuring face of his finitude; in it, death is endlessly repeated, but it is also exorcized; and although it ceaselessly reminds man of the limit that he bears within him, it also speaks to him of that technical world that is the armed, positive, full form of his finitude." Michel Foucault, *Naissance de la clinique*, 6th ed. (Paris: Quadrige/Presses universitaires de France, 2000 [1963]), 201–02. English excerpt from home.ku.edu.tr/~mbaker/cshs503/foucaultclinic.pdf. Without stating it explicitly, Foucault is repeating an idea put forward by Georges Canguilhem.
2 *Rieff, The Triumph of the Therapeutic. Uses of Faith after Freud.*

https://doi.org/10.1515/9783110638950-004

anced and in fact identical. When health is salvation, it becomes easy to take the next step and to theorize perfect health, in other words to seek immortality.[3]

This unprecedented situation in Western history has given medicine social and symbolic prestige, and actual power, in our individual and collective lives, whether our daily lives or the political life of the State.[4] Medical practice has, whether we want it to or not, become a locus of power. This includes biomedicine's socially-recognized capacity to define what an ideally healthy life is. Obviously, not all the healthcare professions enjoy the same prestige or symbolic capital as medicine. However, these internal differences do not change the fact that healthcare institutions have acquired enormous capital in Western societies and have become, *nolens volens*, institutions of "salvation".

Through the importance placed by Western culture on health and on healthcare institutions, the biomedical sciences have a determining influence over the way in which the human body and mind, and their integrity, are considered. An overview, even superficial, of modern medical history in the West reveals that the biomedical sciences, like King Midas in Greek mythology, transform everything they touch and, along with the technical applications they make possible, have transformed several areas of care: approaches to death, lifestyles, care practices, etc. Not only do they transform practices, but they have also changed human representations of the fundamental realities that regulate life and death. It is possible to suggest that the biomedical sciences and the care technologies they engender have become a key agent of change in our culture, and to a remarkable anthropological degree. We can look at two examples: representations of health, and representations of death.[5]

---

3 Céline Lafontaine, *La société post-mortelle: la mort, l'individu et le lien social à l'ère des technosciences* (Paris: Seuil, 2008); Lucien Sfez, *L'utopie de la santé parfaite*, Colloque de Cerisy (Paris: Presses universitaires de France, 2001).

4 According to the WHO's 2016 statistics, health spending represented an average of 10% of the gross domestic product of its 39 member countries, from 5.2% in Turkey, the lowest figure, to 16.9% in the United States. Canada was at 10.1%. Source: OCDE, "Statistiques de l'OCDE sur la santé 2016." http://oecd.org/fr/els/systemes-sante/base-donnees-sante.htm. As a comparison, military spending by central governments represented in 2015, an average of 2.28% of GDP, with the US spending 5.6%. Source: Banque mondiale, "Dépenses militaires (% du PIB)." http://donnees.banquemondiale.org/indicateur/MS.MIL.XPND.GD.ZS.

5 Of course, any representation of health also includes a representation of sickness. The same applies to representations of death, which affect the meaning of the term "life".

3.1 Health

Health and its corollary, sickness, are realities that are first and foremost culturally determined[6]. As mentioned by anthropologist Maurice Godelier, "each culture makes rules to translate an internal change, a painful alteration, or a disability experienced by an individual, into symptoms. And each culture makes rules to link symptoms to causes, thereby determining the nature of the actions taken with respect to a suffering person, whether by a great surgeon or an African therapist."[7] From an anthropological point of view, biomedical science and biomedical practice are an integral part of a given culture. Despite their claims to directly address the manifestations of sickness or health, they cannot escape from the culture they have helped define, in particular since the emergence of the "therapy society". In my opinion it would be better to call this the "care society", given the fact that care has acquired the value of a "total social fact", to use the apt expression coined by Marcel Mauss.

Based on the findings of the anthropology of healthcare, it appears that biomedical sciences and practices play a significant cultural role in shaping our representations of health. It would be extremely interesting to examine the successive representations of health that have marked the history of Western medicine, but for the purposes of this book, I will limit my review to a few key moments from the period of medicine marked by what historians have called the experimental revolution.[8]

Although, for a long time, the notion of health was strongly dependent on the Hippocratic theory of the balance of humours,[9] this was clearly no longer the case in the 19th century. The famous French physiologist Claude Bernard stated that there was no discontinuity between a healthy and a pathological state. Sickness was an abnormal condition, a functional derangement of the corresponding normal state.[10] Each pathological state was matched by a healthy

6 Johannes Bircher, "Towards a Dynamic Definition of Health and Disease," *Medicine, Health Care and Philosophy* 8 (2005): 335.
7 Maurice Godelier, "Maladie et santé selon les sociétés et les cultures," in *Maladie et santé selon les sociétés et les cultures*, ed. Jean-Pierre Dozon et al. (Paris: Presses universitaires de France, 2011): 19.
8 Jean-Charles Sournia, *Histoire de la médecine*, Sciences humaines et sociales (Paris: La Découverte, 1997), 209–17; Maurice Tubiana, *Histoire de la pensée médicale. Les chemins d'Esculape*, Champs (Paris: Flammarion, 1995), 199–202.
9 Jackie Pigeaud, *Poétiques du corps. Aux origines de la médecine* (Paris: Les Belles Lettres, 2009), 7–8.
10 Claude Bernard, *Principes de médecine expérimentale* (Paris: Quadrige/Presses universitaires de France, 2008 [1947]), 138–40.

state, which could be regained. According to Bernard, the passage from a healthy state to a morbid state, and vice versa, could be explained by the intrinsic link between sickness and health, a link based on the quantitative variability of human bodily functions.

This physiological discourse on health and sickness, based on the experimental scientific method, did not prevent the creation of representations that depended more on the experience of patients. For example, in 1936 physician René Leriche proposed a definition of health as "life lived in the in the silence of the organs."[11] Although Leriche supported Bernard's physiological representation of sickness, his medical interest in pain,[12] an ultimately individual experience, clearly influenced his way of considering health, relying not on a "scientific" definition but on individual bodily experience. This bias was adopted by the World Health Organization in its definition of health, and I will come back to it later.

In contrast with, and in some senses in opposition to, Claude Bernard's approach, physician and philosopher Georges Canguilhem presented sickness and health not as two states separated by a quantitative difference, but as two states differing qualitatively from the environment in which an organism lives. The key concept used to designate the activity of a living being, whether healthy or sick, is normativity, which Canguilhem defines as the capacity of a living organism to institute norms, in other words an ability to combat whatever injures or attacks it. Biological normativity is the "spontaneous effort [of a living being] of defense and struggle against all that is of negative value",[13] directed against whatever threatens its integrity. This leads Canguilhem to write that "Disease is still a norm of life but it is an inferior norm in the sense that it tolerates no deviation from the conditions in which it is valid, incapable as it is of changing itself into another norm. The sick living being [...] has lost his normative capacity, the capacity to establish other norms in other conditions. [...] disease is not a variation on the dimension of health; it is a new dimension of life."[14] Health and sickness

---

11 Olivier Bézy, "Quelques commentaires à propos de la célèbre formule de René Leriche: 'La santé c'est la vie dans le silence des organes'," *La revue lacanienne*, no. 3 (2009). Georges Canguilhem, *Le normal et le pathologique* (Paris: Quadrige/Presses universitaires de France, 1966), 52–60.

12 Leriche published a book about pain at the end of World War I. The following quote is attributed to him: "The study of pain leads to a form of medicine that focuses on humanity in all its actions", in Bézy, "Quelques commentaires à propos de la célèbre formule de René Leriche: 'La santé c'est la vie dans le silence des organes'": 47.

13 Canguilhem, *Le normal et le pathologique*, 81.

14 Canguilhem, *Le normal et le pathologique*, 119–20.

are therefore manifestations of balance with the environment, the former being optimal and the latter sub-optimal.

The "subjective turn" in definitions of health was consecrated by the definition drawn up and included in the founding constitution of the World Health Organization (WHO) in 1948: "Health is a state of complete physical, mental and social well-being and not merely the absence of disease or infirmity."[15] The WHO definition presents a holistic view of health that is not solely quantitative, since the notion of wellbeing that lies at the heart of the definition inevitably includes a component of personal assessment. Against the background of the post-World War II period (and the crimes against humanity perpetrated by Nazi physicians) and the Cold War, this tacit emphasis on the eminently personal dimension of the definition of health resonated strongly with the new focus on human rights and the need to affirm, in a clear and strong voice, the inviolability of human beings and respect for their inalienable rights. Since then, the deficiencies of the definition have been exposed: first, it is unachievable in a world with limited resources; second, it is closer to a definition of happiness than of health; and third, it opens the door to a medicalization of happiness thanks to the close association of happiness and health.[16]

These arguments lead to the question of the social consequences of representations of health. One of the crucial issues of healthcare systems in the Western world is their economic viability. As we mentioned above, health expenditure has been increasing constantly in the OECD countries since the middle of the 20th century, increasing the precariousness of the various (private or public) mechanisms put in place to finance healthcare delivery. This situation cannot be unconnected with representations of health, and the connection works both ways. This is why one current theoretical trend is to reflect on a notion or concept of health that takes into account the context of financial and institutional precariousness. Bircher, for example, proposes a "dynamic" definition of sickness and health based on the holistic standpoint of the WHO definition, while qualifying the optimal state represented by health. As a result, the concepts of health and sickness can be described as follows: "Health is a dynamic state of wellbeing

---

15 Preamble to the Constitution of the World Health Organization as adopted by the International Health Conference, New York, 19 June – 22 July 1946; signed on 22 July 1946 by the representatives of 61 States (Official Records of the World Health Organization, no. 2, p. 100) and entered into force on 7 April 1948, WHO, "Preamble to the Constitution of the World Health Organization." https://www.who.int/about/fr/.
16 Rodolfo Saracci, "The World Health Organisation Needs to Reconsider Its Definition of Health," *British Medical Journal* 314, no. 7091 (1997). We will see later how the same criticism can also be levelled at the close link made between health and spiritual wellbeing.

characterized by a physical, mental and social potential, which satisfies the demands of a life commensurate with age, culture, and personal responsibility. If the potential is insufficient to satisfy these demands the state is disease."[17] The following observations can be made: 1) the focus is on potential rather than a holistic state; 2) the plasticity of this potential varies depending on the individual concerned and his or her background; 3) the potential is related to the requirements of the background.[18]

To complete this summary investigation of changes in the concept of health in recent biomedical thought, we must also mention the effort made to integrate the spiritual question into the notion of health itself. The 6th Global Conference on Health Promotion was organized by the WHO and the Ministry of Public Health, Thailand, and held in Bangkok in 2005, bringing together a group of international experts. The final document stipulates that

> the enjoyment of the highest attainable standard of health is one of the fundamental rights of every human being without discrimination. Health promotion is based on this critical human right and offers a positive and inclusive concept of health as a determinant of the quality of life *and encompassing mental and spiritual well-being*. Health promotion is the process of enabling people to increase control over their health and its determinants, and thereby improve their health. It is a core function of public health and contributes to the work of tackling communicable and noncommunicable diseases and other threats to health.[19]

Drawing explicitly on the human rights discourse and making health and, therefore, spiritual wellbeing public health issues, the Bangkok consensus presents a view of health that also aligns with the *idées-forces* embodied in the definition of health adopted by the WHO in 1948. Health is not limited to physiological functions, but also includes the psychological, social and now spiritual aspects of human life. I will go no further here, since I will deal in detail with this holistic concept of health, and the link with spirituality, in the next chapter. For now, it is sufficient to say that the most recent approaches to the notion of health in medical thought incorporate concerns that open it up to dimensions of human life that were not part of the modern vision of medicine, health and sickness. This conception of health contrasts with that of modern medicine described with

---

17 Bircher, "Towards a Dynamic Definition of Health and Disease": 336.
18 Honouring, without naming them, the concerns raised by Canguilhem, in particular considering health and sickness in terms of normativity.
19 WHO, *La Charte de Bangkok pour la promotion de la santé à l'heure de la mondialisation*, (2005), http://www.who.int/healthpromotion/conferences/6gchp/BCHP_fr.pdf. 2. [Emphasis mine]. English excerpt from *The Bangkok Charter for Health Promotion in a Globalized World* https://www.who.int/healthpromotion/conferences/6gchp/hpr_050829_%20BCHP.pdf?ua=1

such accuracy by Foucault in *Naissance de la clinique* when, seeking to determine "the conditions of possibility of medical experience in modern times",[20] he states that for the science of medicine that emerged in the early 19th century, pathology was considered to be "an organic reaction to an irritating agent"[21] and that "a medicine of pathological reactions [was] a structure of experience that dominated the nineteenth century, and, to a certain extent, the twentieth."[22]

The notion of health is therefore variable and we have seen how changes in medical culture, brought about first by the biological sciences and then by the incorporation of a holistic concept of care, have changed the very idea of what we think of as health.

3.2 Death

Contemporary representations of death have already been subjected to widespread scientific scrutiny. My objective, here, is to show how the transformation of medical culture has changed contemporary conceptions and representations of death.

If, as stated by sociologist Michel Castra "the conditions of death changed significantly during the 20th century [...] reflecting changes in medical techniques and the movement towards a specialization of medicine",[23] the impact of the changes can also be observed in two key areas: in their clinical aspect, the criteria for death, and in their symbolic aspect, the desocialization of death.

3.2.1 Death: clinical aspects

Medical resuscitation technologies, developed in the mid- century, have had a significant impact on representations of death. Now that a body can be kept alive by assisted hydration and ventilation, even in the absence of higher-order cerebral functions, the question of how to determine the exact moment of death has arisen, in particular given the development of organ transplantation technologies and techniques. This phenomenon is discussed by Céline Lafon-

20 Foucault, *Naissance de la clinique*, xv.
21 Foucault, *Naissance de la clinique*, 194.
22 Foucault, *Naissance de la clinique*, 196.
23 Michel Castra, *Bien mourir. Sociologie des soins palliatifs*, ed. Serbe Paugam, Le Lien social (Paris: Presses universitaires de France, 2003), 23.

taine in *La société post-mortelle* in a chapter entitled "Les nouvelles frontières de la mort" ("the new frontiers of death").[24] It is important to note that this reconceptualization is closely linked to the definition of new criteria for clinical death, based on cerebral death, that are not those used over many centuries by the medical world. Previously, the passage from life to death occurred "instantly" based on clear physical criteria: cardiac arrest, respiratory arrest, or a lack of reaction to pain stimuli. After a period of "dying" of varying duration depending on the illness involved, death occurred "almost" instantly. Technological progress in the clinical sciences stretched this "moment" into a "process", changing the temporal register of death. Instead of being instantaneous, it now took place over time. As a result, the criteria for death became: a total lack of response to stimuli, including the most painful; a total absence of movement and spontaneous respiration; the complete disappearance of all reflexes.[25] The new criteria distinguish between cerebral and corporeal death, forming a "disembodied" view of the subject[26], in other words one in which subjectivity is independent of the body. These new criteria appear to surreptitiously re-introduce a dualistic, body/spirit vision of the human being. They re-establish a conception in which the subject has a body ("I have a body"), in contrast to a phenomenological approach that emphasizes the firmly embodied condition of human life ("I am a body").

3.2.2 Death: symbolic aspects

The effects of the technological revolution on the definition of death combine with a more long-standing process in which medical practice has taken control over the present-day conditions for dying. This is described by historian Philippe Ariès in his research into the conditions for dying in the Western world. He describes a phenomenon he calls the "medicalization of death", whose origin he places in the mid-19th century.[27] This expression should not be understood as

---

24 Lafontaine, *La société post-mortelle: la mort, l'individu et le lien social à l'ère des technosciences*, 69–96.
25 Lafontaine, *La société post-mortelle: la mort, l'individu et le lien social à l'ère des technosciences*, 79. Lafontaine cites philosopher Anne Fagot-Largeault, *Les causes de la mort. Histoire naturelle et facteurs de risques* (Paris: Vrin, 1989), 20.
26 Lafontaine, *La société post-mortelle: la mort, l'individu et le lien social à l'ère des technosciences*, 82.
27 Philippe Ariès, *L'homme devant la mort 2. La mort ensauvagée*, Points Histoire 83 (Paris: Seuil, 1977), 269–311.

meaning a techno-scientific taking of control which, as I explained above, is a later meaning that is only valid from the mid-20th century onwards. Instead, it refers to a change in the culture of death in the Western world, introduced by the growing role and prestige of medicine in the modern age. Ariès describes two dimensions that help make death a medical and private, even hidden, reality, where previously it had been a "social and public fact".[28]

First, physicians gained the power to decide whether or not to reveal their state to patients[29] as religion and priests gradually lost their role as regulators of the process of dying. Second, death no longer occurred in the home, but in hospital[30]. This trend gained pace along with increased medical intervention at the end of a patient's life, but stabilized with the arrival of palliative care in the late 1960s. However, it is important to emphasize that death remained "institutionalized", in the sense that most people still died in a care facility, away from home. As a result, death was "desocialized" to a certain extent, since it was increasingly removed from the proximity and social circle of the patient's everyday life.

In short, after death was attracted into medicine's sphere of influence, the conditions of death changed radically in terms of time, space and perception. In terms of time, death was no longer the rapid extinguishment of life, but a drawn-out and slow process. Although it is still a shock to find out that our own death is imminent, the fact remains that except in unusual circumstances the process itself now takes longer than before the advent of techno-scientific medicine. The spatial setting, previously family and social, has become a "private" space in a care facility. Death, which was seen as a natural occurrence, has become a process strewn with technological artifice. Of course, since the dawn of human time, death has always been lived within a cultural matrix, meaning that it was part of the culture and surrounded by cultural practices. Until modern times, this cultural matrix considered death as a natural process. Since the advent of the biomedical techno-sciences death is increasingly seen as a non-natural phenomenon, and even as a phenomenon with entirely artificial components. The process of dying has been integrated into the sphere of human actions, where it is no longer seen as a strictly natural occurrence.

---

28 Ariès, *L'homme devant la mort 2. La mort ensauvagée*, 269.

29 Ariès, *L'homme devant la mort 2. La mort ensauvagée*, 270 – 77.

30 Ariès, *L'homme devant la mort 2. La mort ensauvagée*, 280 – 81. Lafontaine, *La société post-mortelle: la mort, l'individu et le lien social à l'ère des technosciences*, 31– 33.

3.3 Intermediate conclusion

These two brief excursions show how biomedical thought and practice have influenced the contemporary representations of health and death. We have seen how the biomedical viewpoint is a powerful agent for cultural change, and a powerful agent for the establishment of an order or "structure" on which representations of health and death are placed and take the form dictated by biomedicine. Yes, our representations, previously embedded in centuries-old and mainly religious traditions, are now formatted to a certain extent by biomedical thought and practice. The weight of the traditions was not great enough to prevent the metamorphosis. Should we consider the possibility that the spiritual experience will not be able to escape the same attraction, once it becomes a focus of biomedicine? Can this area of human life "resist" the transforming power of contemporary biomedicine? Is medicalization to be the fate of everything touched by biomedicine? Will spirituality emerge unscathed from its contact with biomedicine?

I will leave these questions unanswered for now, since the next chapter will contribute more elements to the debate.

First, though, the topics we have just explored must be placed along one of the structuring axes of biomedical thought and practices, namely the quest for order and its corollary, harmony.

3.4 The quest for order and harmony

Medical research and practice are founded on the idea that order exists in this world along with an optimal way for the functioning of all things, and that it can be rationally and scientifically identified. Physicians in the Hippocratic tradition thought that health resulted from a perfect qualitative and quantitative balance between the four constituent liquids mixed within the human body. This is the well-known ancient theory of the balance of humours. Imbalance, resulting from the separation or isolation of any of these physiological fluids, could endanger health.[31] The optimal order, in this case, lay within the body, but according to Pigeaud the order of the humours was, for the Ancients, analogous to the order that governed the universe. Here, we can see the origin of the Western medical idea of an intimate and close association between order, harmony—via the notion of balance—and normal physiological functions.

---

31 Pigeaud, *Poétiques du corps. Aux origines de la médecine*, 7–8.

This tradition was maintained during the Renaissance. Since *On the Fabric of the Human Body*, the *opus magnum* of Andreas Vesalius (1514–1564) in which he posits that "anatomical study [...] must be considered the solidest foundation of the medical art and the beginning of the constitution",[32] the question of order and harmony has played a central role. Once again according to Pigeaud, Vesalus was convinced, like his master from ancient times, Galen,[33] that anatomy revealed the aesthetic and functional perfection of the human being: "One cannot remain unmoved by this strength of Vesalius' work. Nature, the *Opifex*, the *Creator*, and the *Conditor* put together piece by piece, and solved problem after problem, to make a perfect man and perfect woman, designed to function perfectly, and that could only be updated for specific reasons."[34] And this harmonious perfection was "charming" and "pleasing" because it matched that of the universe itself. Addressing the Emperor Charles V, for whom *On the Fabric of the Human Body* was intended, Vesalius predicted that he would be "delighted at times by the contemplation of the fabric of the most perfect of all creatures; so also you must take pleasure in consideration of the dwelling place and implement of the immortal soul, since, due to its remarkable correspondence to the world in many of the names, it was called a 'little world' by the ancients."[35]

This attitude towards the human body, its internal harmony and its resonance with the world of which it forms a part, was still conveyed by scholars in the 20th century, for example in the work of British endocrinologist Ernest Starling. He ended a famous talk, *The Wisdom of the Body*, given in 1923 to the Royal College of Physicians as a *Harveian Oration*, with the following words:

> In our childhood most of us learnt that suffering and death came into the world through sin. Now, when as physicians we stand on the other side of good and evil, we know that the sin for which man is continuously paying the penalty is not necessarily failure to comply with some one or other of the rough tribal adjustments to the environment, which we call morality, but is always and in every case ignorance or disregard of the immutable working of the forces of Nature which is being continually revealed to us by scientific investigation. In spite of the marvellous increase in knowledge, to some aspects of which I have drawn your attention, suffering is still widespread amongst us. Only by following out the

---

32 André Vésale, *La fabrique du corps humain*, ed. Claire Ambroselli, La fabrique du corps humain (Arles: Actes Sud/INSERM, 1987[1543]), 29.

33 Jackie Pigeaud, "L'esthétique de Galien," *Mètis. Anthropologie des mondes grecs anciens* 6, no. 1–2 (1991): 7–42. Jackie Pigeaud, *L'art et le vivant*, nrf essais (Paris: Gallimard, 1995), 27–153.

34 Pigeaud, *L'art et le vivant*, 168. The Latin terms mean: maker (*opifex*), creator (*creator*), founder or preserver (*conditor*).

35 Vésale, *La fabrique du corps humain*, 49.

injunction of our great predecessor,[36] —to search out and study the secrets of Nature by way of experiment—can we hope to attain to a comprehension of "the wisdom of the body and of the understanding of the heart", and thereby to the mastery of disease and pain which will enable us to relieve the burden of mankind.[37]

This quotation reveals several different facets of the sapiential view of medicine. First, it is based on worldly wisdom, rather than a religious interpretation of the human condition. It could even be said that by taking a position against a moral judgment on suffering, Starling is moving clearly way from a providential conception of the way in which the world is organized. It is Nature that, in his view, acts as the organizing principle for harmony, which is shattered by illness. Next, it is by the modern means of experimentation that human beings will be able to discover the secrets that Nature seems to want to hide. However, this quest has two inter-related objectives. The technical objective of controlling sickness and suffering, thanks to experimental research, serves a humanist, and even moral objective: to assuage the pain and suffering inflicted on human beings by sickness.

This is the message that French physician and philosopher Philippe Meyer, who supports a resolutely materialist understanding of human nature and phenomena, relays today when he highlights the correspondence between the internal constitution of the living world and the cognitive capacity of the human spirit to understand this order: "the living world can be seen as a material whole determined by a form of internal cohesion that is specific to it and accessible to human reasoning."[38]

The medical mindset,[39] even under the auspices of science, is shaped by the idea of an optimal order that needs to be discovered, a task accessible to the human mind when guided by the experimental scientific method, and a set of relations between human beings and the universe that, when functioning optimally, constitute health.

These few historical examples show that, in various ways, the quest for order has been a constant feature of the medical mindset. However, what distinguishes

---

36 Starling was referring to British physician and anatomist William Harvey (1578 – 1657), who gave the first experimental description of the circulation of blood by the heart.
37 Christiane Sinding, "Une utopie médicale," in *Une utopie médicale La Sagesse du corps par Ernest Starling*, ed. Christiance Sinding, La fabrique du corps humain (Arles: Acte Sud/INSERM, 1989): 95 – 97.
38 Philippe Meyer, *Philosophie de la médecine* (Paris: Bernard Grasset, 2000), 141 – 42.
39 The expression is borrowed from Pigeaud, *Poétiques du corps. Aux origines de la médecine*, IX.

the biomedical culture of the present day from that of previous eras is a repositioning of biomedicine with respect to its centuries-old role.

3.5 From auxiliary to auxiliatory medicine

Medicine in the 20th century was no longer the medicine practised in previous times. Thanks to technoscience it was no longer simply an auxiliary element in the natural healing process, but rather a process that took over when the natural healing process proved unable to restore health. Medicine came to "the assistance" of a healing process that was insufficient in itself, becoming auxiliatory. Discussing this change in the representation of medicine, historian Christiane Sinding wrote about the idea of medical intervention: "We can no longer rely on the *vix* (sic) *medicatrix naturae*, the classic healing power of nature, the true wisdom of the body, which until the second half of the 19th century was simply given a helping hand according to Hippocratic principles; we must now identify its deficiencies and remedy them, we must get around and even combat it: this is the shift that lies behind the all-conquering medicine of the 20th century."[40] The 20th century saw a shift in the centre of gravity, from the previous restorative medicine[41] to a health-creating form of medicine.

This change, which reflects an undeniable increase in power, was in fact the establishment of a new practical order and a new relationship with the real world. Medicine was no longer limited to a supporting role, but took responsibility for the gaps in the natural healing process and searched for techniques and practices that could produce healing or attenuate symptoms. The development of a therapeutic "arsenal" against infectious disease and cancer in the 20th century are clear examples of the new practical order that became established. It could even be described as a Promethean form of medicine, one that no longer looks to an overriding order and no longer respects the limits set, whether by an otherworldly figure such as Providence or a worldly figure such as the *vis medicatrix naturae*.

The transforming power that characterizes biomedicine affects all the "objects" it touches. It integrates them into its structure and into the order it produces and creates. Like "health" or "death", the spiritual experience during illness has also been integrated into the new order of auxiliatory medicine and has been

40 Sinding, "Une utopie médicale": 31.
41 Claire Ambroselli, Anne Fagot-Largeault, and Christiane Sinding, "Avant-propos," in *La fabrique du corps humain* (Arles: Actes sud/INSERM, 1987): 14.

shaped by its ways of thinking and acting. The next chapter will examine this aspect in more detail.

4 Sapientialization of the spiritual question

What we have presented as a postulate must now be proved. This chapter will be devoted to an explanation of how the spiritual experience during illness has been received into contemporary clinical culture.

4.1 Preliminary remarks

Before looking specifically at the mechanism of sapientialization, two key elements of vocabulary need to be clarified. This will, at the same time, help explain how the healthcare world has opened up to the spiritual dimension of illness.

4.1.1 Institutionalization

The new openness to the spiritual experience in the clinical world is an example of the institutionalization process, when an institution, in this case a healthcare institution, takes charge of a human reality. Every institutionalization process has two interdependent dimensions. The first is the creation of system of actions, coordinated to varying degrees, that a single player would not be able to perform alone. For example, a pain management protocol, in the form of a decision-making algorithm or clinical guideline, is a coordinated system of actions that assigns clinical responsibilities within a team or between departments. In this sense, institutionalization is a process that enables actions and makes them permanent. The second dimension is that this automatically leads to a "formatting" of the realities targeted by the institution's operations. We can go back to the example of the pain management protocol, in which pain is primarily perceived in terms of its somatic manifestations. Pain is seen as a clinical problem, and not as a philosophical or theological problem, even if philosophy and theology can provide some insights. The diagnostic action is not speculation about the meaning of pain as part of the human experience. In other words, the clinical protocol for pain management coordinates actions and, at the same time, indicates which aspects of the pain experience will be addressed by the care team. The protocol provides an example of how the institution makes complex actions possible while aiming them in a specific direction.

If we leave the biomedical world for a moment to look at the question in more general terms, we see that institutionalization of the spiritual experience

https://doi.org/10.1515/9783110638950-005

is a relatively frequent occurrence. Western history offers many examples of institutionalization of the spiritual experience, in particular in the history of the Christian churches, through the birth, development and, in some cases, death of spiritual families. This rich and complex story, in which various spiritual influences interweave, also shows that the spiritual experience is not easy to structure in an institutional environment. As an interruption of everyday life, the spiritual experience may be supported by social structures—the long-standing presence of monastic religious communities and mendicant orders demonstrates this—but may also resist institutional structures. Spiritual groups claiming evangelical inspiration and struggling against the ecclesial and political structures of their time[1] or instances of reform within institutionalized spiritual groups leading to schisms[2] are common in the history of the Christian churches. The question here is not to award praise or blame to various groups, but to highlight the fact that although the spiritual experience can be institutionalized, the process always occurs in a state of tension between institutional structures and experiential effervescence.

4.1.2 The spiritual experience during illness

The second expression that requires clarification is the one I have chosen to label the focus of my research: the "spiritual experience during illness". I prefer it to other terms such as "spirituality" or "inner life" for the four reasons set out below.

First, it is open-ended and does not refer to a single group within a health-care institution. The spiritual question resonates at several different levels and, although we spontaneously think of the experience of people who are sick, it is worth aiming for a broader view. It has long been recognized that illness does not affect just the sick, but also their relatives and the members of the care team once the sick person is admitted to a healthcare institution and becomes a "patient". This, in fact, is one of the reasons why the medical bio-psycho-social model for dealing with illness was proposed in the 1970s, to ensure consideration for the effects of a person's illness on the members of that person's networks

---

1 The movements involving German peasants in the 15th and 16th centuries, and especially that of Thomas Muntzer, illustrate this form of resistance, which may include violence.
2 Key examples are the internal reforms of Western Christian monasticism since the founding of the Benedictines, and the diversification of the Franciscan spiritual family into several different branches.

of relationships. From this point of view, the circle of people affected by an illness is not limited to the person who is ill.

The second target group is made up of caregivers. The fact that clinical culture is opening up to the spiritual experience is due, in large part, to the interest shown by caregivers in all professional areas. The spiritual experience of caregivers can be triggered by two types of situations. The first is the situation faced by many people working in palliative care when they start to wonder about life, death, the meaning of life, etc., as they look inwards as a result of the clinical situations they encounter.[3] Spending time with patients and their families, listening to their questions about the meaning of life and illness, can lead caregivers to ask themselves similar questions and to live their own spiritual experience. The second situation is connected to the ups and downs of their professional life,[4] for example during their adaptation to difficult working conditions or periods of professional burnout, which lead them to question the meaning of care practices and even the foundations of their professional commitment. In both cases, however, their personal spirituality is at stake because, for caregivers, it is one of the motivating forces for beginning, or continuing, a career in a care profession. Caregivers who provide care in institutions in which the clinical culture is open to the spiritual question may begin, themselves, to question and explore a spiritual horizon or dimension in their professional or personal lives.

---

3 Dana Bjarnason, "Nursing, religiosity, and end-of-life care: interconnections and implications," *Nursing Clinics of North America* 44, no. 4 (2009); Maria E. Boero et al., "Spirituality of health workers: a descriptive study," *Int J Nurs Stud* 42, no. 8 (2005); Mayara G. Camargos et al., "Understanding the Differences Between Oncology Patients and Oncology Health Professionals Concerning Spirituality/Religiosity: A Cross-Sectional Study," *Medicine* (Baltimore) 94, no. 47 (2015); Carmen G. Loiselle and Michelle M. Sterling, "Views on death and dying among health care workers in an Indian cancer care hospice: balancing individual and collective perspectives," *Palliat Med* 26, no. 3 (2012); Edwin J. Pugh et al., "A profile of the belief system and attitudes to end-of-life decisions of senior clinicians working in a National Health Service Hospital in the United Kingdom," *Palliat Med* 23, no. 2 (2009).
4 Terri A. Cavaliere et al., "Moral distress in neonatal intensive care unit RNs," *Adv Neonatal Care* 10, no. 3 (2010); Jean-F. Desbiens and Lise Fillion, "Coping strategies, emotional outcomes and spiritual quality of life in palliative care nurses," *Int J Palliat Nurs* 13, no. 6 (2007); Wendy Duggleby, Dan Cooper, and Kelly Penz, "Hope, self-efficacy, spiritual well-being and job satisfaction," *J Adv Nurs* 65, no. 11 (2009); Devinder Kaur, Murali Sambasivan, and Naresh Kumar, "Effect of spiritual intelligence, emotional intelligence, psychological ownership and burnout on caring behaviour of nurses: a cross-sectional study," *J Clin Nurs* 22, no. 21–22 (2013); Cynda H. Rushton et al., "Burnout and Resilience Among Nurses Practicing in High-Intensity Settings," *Am J Crit Care* 24, no. 5 (2015); Jinsun Yong et al., "Effects of a spirituality training program on the spiritual and psychosocial well-being of hospital middle manager nurses in Korea," *J Contin Educ Nurs* 42, no. 6 (2011).

Last, the potential effect that consideration for the spiritual experience during sickness may have on institutions themselves cannot be ignored.[5] Several stakeholders see this as an opportunity to transform the medical culture, focused on technoscience, and the institutional culture, focused on efficiency and efficacy, since the idea of care is extended beyond considerations of technical efficaciousness, economic cost-effectiveness and managerial efficiency.

In short, the expression "spiritual experience during illness" applies to everyone involved, directly or indirectly, actively or passively, on an occasional or ongoing basis, in the work of a care facility: patients, families, friends, caregivers, other staff members, etc. However, unless otherwise indicated the expression will be used primarily to refer to the spiritual experience of patients.

Second, the expression refers to something real. The word "experience" is based on the idea that a person's spiritual path is reflected in his or her attitudes, feelings, behaviour, ritual or other gestures, words, and special times. The spiritual experience is not based solely on "holding" beliefs that have been deliberately chosen as if part of an intellectual process. "Holding" a belief is an important component of spiritual life, but is not the only manifestation of a spiritual experience.

Third, the spiritual experience has a "public" dimension. The word "experience" distinguishes it from the expression "inner life" that makes a person's spiritual life a strictly private area. Although, of course, our spiritual experience is something inward-looking and intimate that is specific to each individual, we must still recognize that it is expressed in daily life, and in particular in the life of an institution, as highlighted above. The spiritual experience includes a clear institutional and social dimension,[6] whether through the interest taken by shared institutions such as the education system[7] or healthcare system, or

---

5 Frederic C. Craigie, Jr., "Weaving spirituality into organizational life. Suggestions for processes and programs," *Health Prog* 79, no. 2 (1998); Malcolm B. Herring and Jon D. Rahman, "Physicians and spirituality. St. Vincent Indianapolis has a program that encourages spiritual development in doctors," *Health Prog* 85, no. 4 (2004); Rosemary Hume, Sharon Richardt, and Beth Applegate, "Spirituality and work. Indianapolis's Seton Cove Center seeks to integrate spirituality into the workplace," *Health Prog* 84, no. 3 (2003); Jim Letourneau, "Mission Integration and Workplace Spirituality," *Health Prog* 97, no. 2 (2016); Maureen McGuire, "Toward workplace spirituality. St. Louis-based Ascension Health is attending to the "spirit in work"," *Health Prog* 85, no. 6 (2004).
6 Philip F. Sheldrake, *Explorations in Spirituality. History, Theology, dans Social Practice* (New York/Mahwah, NJ: Paulist Press, 2010), 91–156.
7 The United Kingdom's *Education Act, 2002* stipulates that "Every state-funded school must offer a curriculum which is balanced and broadly based and which promotes the spiritual, moral, cultural, mental and physical development of pupils at the school and of society," De-

through the contribution made by the spiritual intuitions promoted by social groups to the transformation of social relationships, institutions, laws, etc. On the topic of the social impact of spiritual intuitions that have left their mark on public life, I can cite the example of various initiatives taken by Canadian believers that led to the establishment of health insurance programs in Canada,[8] or the efforts made by religious groups to welcome refugees at various points in history.[9] To repeat what was mentioned above, the social character of the spiritual experience is closely connected to the institutionalization processes that run through all human groups and all societies. The institutionalization of the spiritual experience can be said to make manifest its social nature.

Last, but not least, the expression "spiritual experience during illness" does not mean that the spiritual experience is "ill" because it occurs during a time of illness. A wide range of spiritual states can be experienced during illness: anger, gratitude towards primary caregivers, anxiety for loved ones, supplications addressed to God, feelings of absurdity, injustice, indignation, plenitude, etc. Patients may find some of these pleasing, while others are harder to accept. Because of the range of spiritual experiences triggered by an illness, it is important, theoretically and practically, not to automatically associate a patient's illness (whether somatic or psychic) with a morbid spiritual state.

---

partment for children schools and families, *Religious education in English schools: Non-statutory guidance 2010*, (Government of United Kingdom, 2010), https://www.gov.uk/government/uploads/system/uploads/attachment_data/file/190260/DCSF-00114 – 2010.pdf. 7. Section 36 of Québec's *Education Act* states that "A school is an educational institution whose object is to provide to the persons entitled thereto under section 1 the educational services provided for by this Act and prescribed by the basic school regulation established by the Government under section 447 and to contribute to the social and cultural development of the community. A school shall, in particular, facilitate the spiritual development of students so as to promote self-fulfilment", in Gouvernement du Québec, *Education Act*, http://www.legisquebec.gouv.qc.ca/en/ShowDoc/cs/I-13.3. Retrieved November 2, 2016.

8 For example, the work of Pastor Thomas (Tommy) Douglas, a federal MP from 1935 to 1944 and 1962 to 1979. He was also Premier of the Canadian province of Saskatchewan from 1944 to 1961. He set up, in his province, the first governmental health insurance program in North America.

9 Examples include the Vietnamese "boat people" who found asylum in Québec in the late 1970s, and the Syrian refugees of 2015 – 2016.

4.2 Conditions for a possible sapientialization of spirituality

As we saw above, sapientialization is the process by which the spiritual experience is received in the biomedical world, with the result that the spiritual experience is reframed as wisdom. It is important to point out right away that this action is performed by a system for thought and action—the biomedical system—and not by isolated individuals. In other words, the phenomenon manifests itself in various ways and includes various factors. Three facilitating factors can be identified, "facilitating" in the sense that, indirectly, they prepare the ground and mindset for receiving the spiritual experience during illness as part of the clinical culture. I present them here in the chronological order of their appearance.

4.2.1 The "invention" of spiritual needs

The expression "spiritual needs" first appeared in the field of nursing in the early 1960s to designate, in a general way, a person's religious experience during a period of illness. Virginia Henderson is credited with "creating" the expression in connection with theories of nursing care.[10] A spiritual need, included in the list of patient needs requiring nursing, was defined as the need felt by a patient to worship according to his or her faith. To meet the need, the nursing action was to provide assistance to allow the patient to worship accordingly.[11] Henderson explained that assistance was an action in response to the patient's right to follow his or her religious beliefs during hospitalization, and that respecting that right was part of basic nursing care.[12] Henderson published her theory at a time when a religious, rite-based framework was used to understand and define the spiritual question. Today, as we will see in this chapter, the semantic field covered by the expression "spiritual need" in nursing theory extends beyond re-

---

10 For the source of Henderson's approach to this notion, see Serena Buchter et al., "Du besoin au désir. La dimension spirituelle dans les soins infirmiers: le point de vue infirmier," in *Besoins spirituels Soin, désir, responsabilités*, ed. Dominique Jacquemin (Bruxelles: Lumen vitae, 2016); Nicolas Vonarx, "De Bronislaw Malinowski à Virginia Henderson: révélation sur l'origine anthropologique d'un modèle de soins infirmiers," *Aporia* 2, no. 4 (2010).

11 Virginia Henderson, *Les principes fondamentaux des soins infirmiers du CII* (Genève: Conseil international des infirmières (CII), 2003 [1960]), 22.

12 Henderson, *Les principes fondamentaux des soins infirmiers du CII*, 51.

ligious rites. This broadening of the notion of spiritual need is motivated and supported by a humanist understanding of spiritual reality.[13]

4.2.2 The institutionalization of palliative care

It is not my goal here to review the emergence, institutionalization and development of palliative care in Western societies from the late 1960s on,[14] but instead to show how palliative care has also left an imprint on the clinical mindset and prepared the ground for consideration for the spiritual experience during illness. The fundamental intuition, first expressed by Cicely Saunders, about the total pain experienced by end-of-life patients is a key element in my argument. Given the limits of curative medicine in end-of-life situations, palliative care emerged as something that could be done when there was nothing else to do. This "doing something" quality of palliative care aimed to mitigate suffering and total pain and to take into account the mental, existential, spiritual and religious issues raised by an advancing cancer and imminent death. In a way, palliative care is a reiteration of the *Ars moriendi*, *Exhortations to the dying person* and other "in contemplation of death" processes defined during the Renais-

---

13 It could be objected, here, that the hospitaller religious communities in the Catholic and Protestant world were already attentive to the spiritual state of their patients, supported by the religious culture of the institutions and good works they established. However, it would be an anachronism to equate the pastoral focus of the hospitaller communities, at a time when medicine and religion cohabited without infringing on each other's fields of action, with the current clinical focus on ensuring that nursing staff identify and, in some cases, accompany patients' spiritual needs. The two situations may appear to be similar at first sight, but the main, and fundamental, difference, lies in the institutional forms developed in response. The pastoral focus of the hospitaller nuns was a step in the process of a clerical, religious and ritual taking in charge of the patients' spiritual needs, while the clinical focus of present-day caregivers is oriented towards a form of spiritual accompaniment that is, in principle, de-traditionalized.

14 David Clark, "From Margins to Center: A Review of the History of Palliative Care in Cancer," *The Lancet*, no. 8 (2007); Stephen R. Connor, "Development of hospice and palliative care in the United States," *Omega (Westport)* 56, no. 1 (2007); Derek Doyle, "Palliative medicine in Britain," *Omega (Westport)* 56, no. 1 (2007); Marie-Louise Lamau and Lucie Hacpille, "Origine et inspiration," in *Manuel de soins palliatifs*, ed. Dominique Jacquemin and Didier de Broucker (Paris: Dunod, 2009); Cicely Saunders, "Caring for cancer," *J R Soc Med* 91, no. 8 (1998); David C. Saunders, "Origins: international perspectives, then and now," *Hosp J 14*, no. 3–4 (1999); Castra, *Bien mourir. Sociologie des soins palliatifs*.

sance.[15] These religious tools were available to laypersons and clerics to deal with the religious and spiritual questions that arise at the end of life. The similarity between palliative care and these older spiritual methods does not lie in their religious content, but in the support provided for the process of dying, which may include spiritual support if the dying person so desires. In short, questions about the meaning of life, death, pain and suffering are likely to be asked at the end of a person's life, and palliative care has created an ideal clinical space where they can be heard and addressed.

4.2.3 A new proposal for a clinical approach to illness

Anyone who comes into extended contact with the care system or the training provided for caregivers will quickly notice that the adjective "biopsychosocial" has become an integral part of the language used in contemporary clinical culture. It designates a key aspect in the way illness is addressed and in the care provided to patients. It means that caregivers must pay attention to the biological, psychological and social repercussions of illness on the life of the patient and the patient's family. This understanding of the scope of care, which has achieved a consensus and today passes without mention, is in fact a relatively recent development in the healthcare world.

In 1977, US psychiatrist George Engel wrote an article for a leading journal, *Science*, called "The Need for a New Medical Model: A Challenge for Biomedicine."[16] In it, he criticized two positions common in psychiatry at the time; the first, that psychiatry should be excluded from medicine and included with the behavioural sciences (such as psychology), and the second, that psychiatry should be aligned with the medical model and limited to the behavioural problems caused by disturbances in the brain's operation.

Engel disagreed with both positions, which shared the same idea of psychiatric illness, reducing it to its biological causes and defining it as a departure from a measurable biological norm.[17] According to Engel, these representations were difficult to apply in the field of psychiatry, since they resulted from the ap-

15 Florence Bayard, *L'art de bien mourir au XVᵉ siècle* (Paris: Presses de l'Université de Paris-Sorbonne, 1999); Érasme, *La préparation à la mort* (Montréal: Éditions Paulines/Apostolat des Éditions, 1976[1533]).
16 Engel, "The need for a new medical model: a challenge for biomedicine".
17 It is important to note that this conception of illness, based on 19th-century positivist science, had already been criticized in the early 1940s by philosopher and physician Georges Canguilhem (cf. chap. 1).

plication of a reductionist model of sickness to its biological component. Engel did not deny that mental illness had a biological component, but did not consider it to be its sole characteristic, rejecting this restricted interpretation and proposing a new medical model that he called biopsychosocial. "To provide a basis for understanding the determinants of disease and arriving at rational treatments and patterns of health care, a medical model must also take into account the patient, the social context in which he lives, and the complementary system devised by society to deal with the disruptive effects of illness, that is, the physician role and the health care system."[18] Engel's proposal was widely discussed, with contributions to the debate from both critics and supporters of his model.[19] What is important here, however, is that the model was adopted relatively quickly in psychiatry and other sectors of medicine, whatever the outcome of the epistemological debates about the relevance and perfectibility of Engel's theory.

The biopsychosocial model "shattered" the biological sciences' stranglehold over the definition of sickness by including cultural, sociological and psychological elements in the debate about the concept. It also helped broaden the spectrum of the interdisciplinary practices used with patients. Other caregivers (nurses, physiotherapists, occupational therapists, etc.) and other care professionals (psychologists, social workers, etc.) could now help make decisions and

---

18 Engel, "The need for a new medical model: a challenge for biomedicine": 132.

19 Rolf H. Adler, "Engel's biopsychosocial model is still relevant today," *Journal of Psychosomatic Research* 67, no. 6 (2009); Ana S. Alvarez, Marco Pagani, and Paolo Meucci, "The clinical application of the biopsychosocial model in mental health: a research critique," *American journal of physical medicine & rehabilitation* 91, no. 13 Suppl 1 (2012); R. Barker Bausell and Brian M. Berman, "Commentary: alternative medicine: is it a reflection of the continued emergence of the biopsychosocial paradigm?," *American journal of medical quality* 17, no. 1 (2002); Tony B. Benning, "Limitations of the biopsychosocial model in psychiatry," *Advances in medical education and practice* 6 (2015); George L. Engel, "How much longer must medicine's science be bound by a seventeenth century world view?," *Psychotherapy and psychosomatics* 57, no. 1–2 (1992); George L. Engel, "From biomedical to biopsychosocial. Being scientific in the human domain," *Psychosomatics* 38, no. 6 (1997); George L. Engel, "From biomedical to biopsychosocial. 1. Being scientific in the human domain," *Psychotherapy and psychosomatics* 66, no. 2 (1997); Giovanni A. Fava and Nicoletta Sonino, "The biopsychosocial model thirty years later," *Psychotherapy and psychosomatics* 77, no. 1 (2008); Alfred M. Freedman, "The biopsychosocial paradigm and the future of psychiatry," *Comprehensive psychiatry* 36, no. 6 (1995); Suzanne R. Karl and Jimmie C. Holland, "The Roots of Psychosomatic Medicine II: George L. Engel," *Psychosomatics* 56, no. 6 (2015); Nicholas Kontos, "Perspective: biomedicine–menace or straw man? Reexamining the biopsychosocial argument," *Academic Medicine* 86, no. 4 (2011); Daniel Richter, "Chronic mental illness and the limits of the biopsychosocial model," *Medicine, health care, and philosophy* 2, no. 1 (1999); Micharl Saraga, Abraham Fuks, and J. Donald Boudreau, "George Engel's Epistemology of Clinical Practice," *Perspectives in biology and medicine* 57, no. 4 (2014).

draw up care plans. The clinical view of illness and its repercussions for individual lives and social life, and the ways of caring for illness, changed with the adoption of the biopsychosocial model. By calling the strictly biological model into question and changing the clinical focus, the biopsychosocial model laid the groundwork for the emergence, twenty-five years later, of a biopsychosocial and spiritual model for illness.

These three events, which occurred relatively recently in the Western world's long history of healthcare, unintentionally helped ensure that the spiritual experience of patients became a "focus" of clinical attention in the late 1980s. The theoretical work of Henderson, Saunders and Engel and the clinical applications it supported made it possible to begin work to prepare mindsets and establish markers to gradually increase caregivers' familiarity with the existential, spiritual and religious questions asked by people dealing with illness. This transformation of mindsets was followed, in practical terms, by the definition of concepts to operationalize the acceptance of the spiritual experience as part of clinical culture. The concepts, generally pragmatic—the definitions of spirituality, spiritual needs and spiritual distress—led, in turn, to various tools to take the spiritual experience during illness into account.

4.3 Definitions of spirituality[20]

A number of authors working on research into the links between spirituality and health have pointed out that there is no consensus concerning the definition of spirituality. Despite this lack of unanimity, an underlying logic can be detected in the various definitions proposed. They are placed along a continuum between two poles, one of which I will describe as humanist and the other as religious. The humanist pole is represented by definitions that consider spirituality to be a strictly human reality, with no connection to any extra-worldly horizon. I use the term extra-worldly advisedly, since even a strictly intra-worldly vision may identify a form of transcendence in immanence, in other words a "connection" between an individual spiritual experience and a horizon of meaning that lies beyond the individual. Nature, the cosmos, or an idealized representation of hu-

---

20 This section is descriptive in nature, and is intended to report on a significant discourse in the Western biomedical world. It is not a definition of spirituality, but a summary of a specific conception of spirituality. I would like to thank Rodrigo Coppe Caldeira for permission to reproduce, here, part of an article published in the journal he edits: Guy Jobin, "Santé, bien-être et spiritualité: une évaluation critique," *Interaçoes – Cultura E Comunidade* 11, no. 20 (2016): 35–36.

manity may all be horizons to which people refer without being tangible manifestations of a level of reality "overhanging" the physical universe in which humanity exists. For example, nurses Murray and Zentner define spirituality as follows:

> In every human being there seems to be a spiritual dimension, a quality that goes beyond religious affiliation, that strives for inspiration, reverence, awe, meaning and purpose, event in those who do not believe in God. The spiritual dimension tries to be in harmony with the universe, strives for answers about the infinite, and comes essentially into focus in terms of emotional stress, physical (and mental illness), loss, bereavement and death.[21]

The religious pole is represented by definitions and representations of spirituality that connect it to a horizon beyond the visible world.

A second axis overlaps the first, since definitions of spirituality may also be placed along a second continuum describing the source of spiritual life. Mirroring the first axis, it has two poles: internal and external. The internal pole indicates that the source of spiritual life is located within each subject, who draws on inner resources to give a meaning to the events that structure his or her life. This way of seeing the source of spiritual life matches another idea, firmly enshrined in the biomedical literature, that human beings are anthropologically spiritual. The external pole includes the discourses that place the source of spirituality outside the individual, in an extra-personal (but not necessarily extra-worldly) "space". Here, spiritual life is seen as belonging to an "order", of whatever nature, or as a gift received from an Other. This is the Christian conception of spiritual life, which is seen as participation, through grace, in divine life.

A large majority of the definitions of spirituality in the biomedical literature belong to the humanist-internal genre. It appears to be the most inclusive and most encompassing, provided, of course, that human beings are anthropologically spiritual and only accidentally (or historically) religious. This postulate constitutes, in itself, a taking of position, clearly assigning the burden of proof to the religious traditions in any discussion of "spirituality". The postulate is also clearly predominant in Western secular culture.

A survey of the various definitions produced by care theorists from various professions reveals several significant recurrences in the humanist-internal definitions of spirituality.[22]

---

21 Ruth Beckmann Murray and Judith Proctor Zentner, *Nursing Concepts for Health Promotion* (London: Prentice Hall, 1989), 259.
22 The following section is largely based on two previous studies: Guy Jobin, *Des religions à la spiritualité: une appropriation biomédicale du religieux dans l'hôpital* (Bruxelles: Lumen vitae, 2012); Guy Jobin, "Êtes-vous en belle santé? Sur l'esthétisation de la spiritualité en bioméde-

Table 1. Representations of spirituality in the healthcare world[23]

Spirituality	Religion
Universal and inherent in human nature	Cultural/historical
Personal, dynamic and authentic quest	Collective and static
Liberty	Constraints (dogmas, authority)
Relationality	Rites-based
Harmony	

4.3.1 Universality and naturality

For the first characteristic, spirituality is seen as an inherent dimension of human nature, one possessed by all members of the human family. As a result, the ability to undergo a spiritual experience is part of the essential fabric of every human being. This means that spirituality is a universal dimension, present in human beings in general and in every human being in particular. The universal nature ascribed to the spiritual experience supports the idea that it exists independently of religious culture and traditions, which are considered to be cultural and historical phenomena that relate to specific times and places. In this optic, spirituality is present everywhere, but exemplified in different traditions. Christian, Jewish, Muslim, Hindu, Buddhist and lay spirituality are branches that, when they are authentic and promote peace and serenity, stem from a single trunk of spirituality common to all humankind. Since spirituality is intrinsically linked to what it means to be human, its natural character is opposed to the cultural, historical and therefore "constructed" or artificial nature of the religious traditions. The biomedical discourse on spirituality relies on the opposing

---

cine," in *Spiritualités et biomédecine Enjeux d'une intégration*, ed. Guy Jobin, Jean-Marc Charron, and Michel Nyabenda (Québec: Presses de l'Université Laval, 2013). The studies were based on the representations of spirituality found in the training handbooks for four health professions: medicine, nursing, clinical psychology, and social work in a healthcare setting.

23 The features attributed by the same sources to religion are placed alongside. This model is similar to what Zinnbauer, Pargament and Scott described, in 1999, as the modern representation of the relationship between spirituality and religion: Brian J. Zinnbauer, Kenneth I. Pargament, Allie B. Scott, "The Emerging Meanings of Religiousness and Spirituality: Problems and Prospects," *Journal of Personality* 67, no. 6 (1999).

terms nature/culture and natural/constructed to distinguish it from religious phenomena.

4.3.2 A personal, dynamic and authentic quest

For care theoreticians, there can be no doubt that a spiritual quest is personal in nature, and at this level they are in phase with contemporary discourses on spirituality. The subjective turn described by a number of sociologists, in other words the subjectivization of belief in Western society, reflects this characteristic.[24] In contrast, the religious experience is seen as a collective phenomenon in which belief is imposed on individuals.

The quest for meaning gives spiritual life its dynamic character, mobilized during times of sickness when the meaning of events and the direction taken by one's life up to that point are called into question or overshadowed. The search for meaning and significance is introduced by questions such as "Why me?", "What have I done to deserve this disease?", etc. These and other questions indicate a search for the meaning of illness if, of course, there is such a meaning. Authenticity is connected to the fact that the meaning sought—a "quest for meaning" expresses the idea that the meaning is not self-evident, and must be searched for and found—is a meaning that is unique to, comes from and speaks of each individual.

The dynamic nature of the quest contrasts with the static nature of the religious traditions, seen as fixed doctrines. The dichotomy between spiritual dynamism and religious stasis is based, in fact, on opposing spirituality as a practical quest with religion as an acceptance of content (with, of course, some practical applications). However, the fundamental contrast is between the practical nature of spirituality and the dogmatic content of religious belief.

4.3.3 Freedom

For care theoreticians, it goes without saying that freedom is both the matrix of and vector for the spiritual quest. The ability to sample and, eventually, select

---

24 Paul Heelas, *Spiritualities of Life. New Age Romanticism and Consumptive Capitalism*, ed. Paul Heelas and Linda Woodhead, Religion and Spirituality in the Modern World (Oxford: Blackwell, 2008); Heelas and Woodhead, *The spiritual revolution: why religion is giving way to spirituality*; Raphaël Liogier, *Souci de soi, conscience du monde: vers une religion globale? [Concern for Oneself, Concern for the World. Toward a Global Religion?]* (Paris: Armand Colin, 2012).

one spiritual tradition, and the ability to select only some elements of a spiritual tradition, are manifestations of contemporary spirituality that indicate freedom, contrasting with the passivity of people who must follow the dogmatic, ethical and ritual rules generally associated with the authority exercised by religious hierarchies.

4.3.4 Relationality

The fourth characteristic of the biomedical understanding of spirituality is "relationality", meaning that the spiritual life during illness is experienced in and through relations with others. Spirituality is seen as a force that causes a sick person (and, in fact, any person) to enter into significant and invigorating relationships with others. In technical terms, spirituality is connected with alterity. A broad range of possibilities exists for the other party in the relationship: from a loved one, Nature or the cosmos, to God or a transcendent figure.

The ability to enter into a relationship with another is a sign (among many others, it must be said) of spiritual vitality. The ability to make contacts, an ability inherent in human life, is interpreted in the healthcare world as having a spiritual dimension or as a sign of a person's spiritual life. Of course, other interpretations are possible, whether psychological, sociological or anthropological. But in the healthcare world, relationality has taken on a central spiritual dimension.

4.3.5 Harmony

The last characteristic of spiritual life is that it is a factor for harmonization in the lives of both individuals and institutions. In other words, the quest for meaning and the dynamic nature of spiritual life are seen as aiming ultimately to achieve a state of harmony. And harmony is seen as a form of adequacy of oneself with oneself or with the various others mentioned previously, a state in which tensions are relieved and gaps filled. Harmony may be accompanied by a feeling of plenitude or wholeness.

These crucial elements create the framework for the effort made to define spirituality in the biomedical literature, whether in research findings or in publications that summarize the state of knowledge at a given point in time, such as training handbooks for the various care professions and related professions. The definition also provides a close fit with contemporary spiritual anthropology, which makes the spiritual experience a reality that "transcends" the religious traditions. To state this in another way, in this definition of spirituality, the spiritual experience may find concrete expression in a religious tradition, but only partially. It may also be manifested in a lay spiritual tradition. Crossing and going beyond the traditional boundaries, spirituality is seen as a fundamental reality because it is an intrinsic attribute of human nature.

Obviously, this definition of spirituality makes each individual the cornerstone of his or her own spiritual life. It does not completely eliminate the various spiritual traditions, but places them on the sidelines, as a bank of resources for the individual quests that are seen as normative.

There is not room here to demonstrate the links between these characteristics and those of contemporary New Age spiritual discourses.[25] It is clear, however, that an influence exists. The biomedical world does not exist in a bubble or as an autarchy. Healthcare institutions are surrounded by the prevailing culture and may act as echo-chambers in which ideas from the ambient culture expand and circulate. However, it is important not to lose sight of the fact that biomedicine has a capacity to impose order that may be directed at these flows of ideas. This will be the focus of the next chapter, which shows how the definition of spirituality used in the biomedical world can become clinically effective. It is not sufficient to provide a definition—it must be made operational if it is to be a relevant tool for guiding clinical thoughts and actions.

---

25 Heelas, *Spiritualities of Life. New Age Romanticism and Consumptive Capitalism*; Heelas and Woodhead, *The spiritual revolution: why religion is giving way to spirituality*; Liogier, *Souci de soi, conscience du monde: vers une religion globale? [Concern for Oneself, Concern for the World. Toward a Global Religion?]*.

5 Pragmatic approaches to sapientialization

What actions, words and clinical tools are used to transpose caregivers' focus on the spiritual experience of patients and family members into the concrete world? How is the focus operationalized in clinical culture? How is the shift from a definition of spirituality to concrete actions supported? These questions lead us to consider pragmatic approaches to the sapientialization of spirituality. I have opted to use the word "pragmatic", which covers a wider semantic field than "practical", because some of the approaches discussed here belong to the theoretical domain, such as the clinical concepts of spiritual need and spiritual distress. However, their theoretical status does not prevent their application in the institutionalization processes that use them.

An analysis of the domain constituted by the clinical focus on spirituality reveals two interpretations of the pragmatic nature of the spiritual experience during illness. The first involves seeing the spiritual experience as a direct focus of care. This interpretation leads to interventions in response to a complaint[1] made by a patient or a patient's family, which is considered by staff to be a spiritual problem that must be remedied. This occurs, for example, when a patient states that he has lost all his markers in his usual spiritual or religious universe. The second interpretation considers the spiritual experience as an adjuvant, or auxiliary resource. In this case the spiritual experience is seen as a resource for the process of recuperation, rehabilitation, recovery or adaptation to the consequences of the sickness, in short as a component in the strategies that aim to improve the patient's clinical condition. I will look at each interpretation in turn.

5.1 The spiritual experience as a direct focus of care

Inevitably, integrating the spiritual experience into the framework for clinical action has made it a direct focus of care. When a reality of human life becomes a focus of care, the result is what an example of what sociologists call the "med-

---

1 The word "complaint" is used here in its clinical, rather than legal, sense. Clinically speaking, a complaint is when a patient explains a feeling of discomfort to a caregiver. It is not the same as a legal complaint, which focuses on the infringement of a right.

https://doi.org/10.1515/9783110638950-006

icalization phenomenon",[2] a complex process in which events in everyday life are "defined and treated as medical problems, usually in terms of illness as disorders."[3] The spiritual life is by no means the only reality of human life to be medicalized, sharing this common ground with conception, childbirth, learning difficulties, declining sexual performance, etc.

In the specific case of the spiritual experience during illness, the medicalization process has so far involved four specific stages: 1) a definition of spirituality (as outlined in the previous chapter); 2) the creation of a biomedical language and concepts to operationalize the definition; 3) the development of tools to measure patients' spiritual state; and 4) the identification of support interventions, and even therapies, to support patients' spiritual experience. The last three stages will be examined in this chapter.

5.1.1 Clinical language about patients' spiritual experience.

Clinical practice is based on action. Any action intended to effect a transformation, in this case in accordance with the goals of medicine and healthcare, must name its target before acting on it. Naming something is not anodyne—it is an act of power. The power to name something is also the power to control it. Giving a name to a reality that is physical or biological, or that exists in the realm of ideas, is a way to impose order and assign a portion of reality to its place in the "order of things". This is why, in the world of healthcare, diagnosis is a key step. Based on a sick person's complaint and his or her symptoms, physicians and caregivers are able to name the state of health or illness they face clinically. They can then act on that state in accordance with the guidelines and recommendations that govern actions in their professional field. This is what applies in the event of physical or mental illness, and it also applies to the spiritual state of sick people in a healthcare environment.

People's spiritual state of people during illness is a reality that is named and assessed to determine if clinical action must be taken. For this purpose, the ref-

---

2 Mélissa Nader, "La médicalisation: concept, phénomène et processus. Émergence, diffusion et reconfigurations des usages du terme médicalisation dans la littérature sociologique" (Université du Québec à Montréal, 2012).

3 Peter Conrad, "Medicalization and Social Control", *Annual Review of Sociology*, vol. 18, 1992, cited in Nader, "La médicalisation: concept, phénomène et processus. Émergence, diffusion et reconfigurations des usages du terme médicalisation dans la littérature sociologique," 86.

erence state is considered to be the state of "spiritual health"[4] experienced by a person whose spiritual experience is close to the ideal state described in biomedical definitions of spirituality.

The concept used to operationalize the biomedical definition of spirituality is spiritual wellbeing. Spiritual wellbeing is used as a yardstick or neutral reference to assess the gap between the person's current and ideal state. For example, one definition of spiritual wellbeing in the healthcare literature is proposed by the North American Nursing Diagnosis Association International (NANDA-I),[5] as "a pattern of experiencing and integrating meaning and purpose in life through connectedness with self, others, art, music, literature, nature, and/or a power greater than one self, which can be strengthened."[6] Spiritual wellbeing therefore encompasses relationships, culture, nature (in the biological and environmental meaning of the term) and a form of transcendence. Spiritual wellbeing induces mental states that become markers or clues that can be observed by caregivers: hope, the meaning and goal of life, peace and serenity, acceptance, submission, love, self pardon, a positive life philosophy, joy, and courage.[7]

This definition positions, and circumscribes, the optimal spiritual state. The gap between this optimal state and the patient's actual situation is considered to be a shortfall that must receive attention from the caregivers, in one way or another. The definition of spiritual wellbeing, which operationalizes the definition of spirituality, clearly has a clinical scope since it determines an optimal level of functionality, a ideal to be attained or re-established.

5.1.1.1 Naming the gap

The clinical language developed to name the gap between the patient's actual situation and the optimal situation is based on two key concepts: spiritual need and spiritual distress. Each names a distinct state.

---

4 For a critical review of the notion of spiritual health, cf. Jobin, "Êtes-vous en belle santé? Sur l'esthétisation de la spiritualité en biomédecine".

5 An international organization whose mission is to facilitate the development, refinement, dissemination and use of a standardized nursing diagnosis terminology. http://www.nanda.org/about-nanda-international.html, retrieved November 22, 2016.

6 NANDA International, "Motivation à améliorer son bien-être spirituel," in *Diagnostics infirmiers Définitions et classification 2012 – 2014* (Issy-les-Moulineaux: Elsevier Masson, 2013): 434.

7 NANDA International, "Motivation à améliorer son bien-être spirituel," 434

Since its appearance in the healthcare literature in the early 1960s, the clinical concept of spiritual need[8] has undergone rapid change. We saw earlier how the founder of a new approach to nursing care in the 20th century, Virginia Henderson, defined the concept of spiritual need.

This was the first time, to the best of my knowledge, that the expression "spiritual need" was used in the language of healthcare, although the religious meaning given by Henderson differed from the meaning assigned by nursing care theoreticians today. In present-day theories of nursing care, spiritual need is defined on the basis of a humanist, rather than a religious, concept. Let us turn, for example, to a definition from a training manual for nursing care, in which Murray, Zentner and Yakimo define spiritual need as "a lack of any factor necessary to establish or maintain a dynamic, personal relationship with God, or a higher being, as defined by the individual."[9] The definition is then related to twenty-one needs in three separate categories, based on the type of relation, as shown in the following table.

Table 2. Spiritual needs according to Murray, Zentner and Yakimo[10]

Needs related to the individual person	Needs related to others	Needs related to the transcendental
Find meaning and purpose	Forgive others	Know there is a God or an ultimate power
Feel useful	Cope with loss of loved ones	Believe God is loving and present
Have vision and hope	Be responsible toward others	Serve and worship God
Be supported in coping with life transitions	Know that and when to give an take	Learn the scriptures or sources inspired by God
Adapt to increasing dependency	Be respected	
Transcend life's challenges		
Maintain personal dignity		

8 This section is an amended version of: Guy Jobin, "Development of the Connection Between Spirituality and Medicine: Historical and Current Issues in Clinics," *Spiritual Care* 6, no. 2 (2017).
9 Ruth Beckmann Murray, Judith Proctor Zentner, and Richard Yakimo, "Spiritual and Religious Influences," in *Health Promotion Strategies Through the Life Span* (Upper Saddle River, NJ: Pearson/Prentice Hall, 2009): 202.
10 Murray, Zentner, and Yakimo, "Spiritual and Religious Influences".

Table 2. Spiritual needs according to Murray, Zentner and Yakimo *(continued)*

Needs related to the individual person	Needs related to others	Needs related to the transcendental
Express feelings		
Have fellowship with others		
Love, serve, and be forgiven		
Have continuity with the past		
Prepare for and accept death		

This list of needs is representative of what is generally presented in the biomedical literature on the topic of spiritual need. Other proposals exist, with varying numbers of identified needs.[11] Despite this difference in number, the proposals all use the term "need" to describe a lack compared to an ideal, optimal state.

A need is a lack that it not necessarily associated with illness, but may be exacerbated when illness causes a person to lose his or her habitual points of reference. However, it is through the identification of a need—whether expressed directly by the patient or interpreted by a member of the care team—that spiritual support can be considered and eventually made available.

The second important diagnostic and clinical term is "spiritual distress", a state described as "the impaired ability to experience and integrate meaning and purpose in life through the person's connections with self, others, art, music, literature, nature, or a power greater than oneself."[12] Also according to NANDA-I, distress is clinically characterized by a set of features classified under various headings:

---

11 For example, Taylor identifies 12 needs, while Craven and Hirnle recognize 7: Ruth F. Craven and Constance J. Hirnle, *Fundamentals of nursing: human health and function*, 5th ed. (Philadelphia: Lippincott Williams & Wilkins, 2007); Carol Taylor, Carol Lillis, and Priscilla LeMone, *Fundamentals of nursing: the art & science of nursing care*, 4th ed. (Philadelphia: Lippincott, 2001).
12 Murray, Zentner, and Yakimo, "Spiritual and Religious Influences": 203.

Table 3. Features of spiritual distress by type of relation[13]

Connections to self	Connections with others	Connections with art, music, literature, nature	Connections with power greater than self
Expresses lack of: — hope — meaning and purpose in life — peace/serenity — acceptance — love — forgiveness of self — courage	Refuses interactions with spiritual leaders	Inability to express previous state of creativity	Inability to pray
Anger	Refuses interactions with friends, family	No interest in nature	Inability to participate in religious activities
Guilt	Verbalizes being separated from their support system	No interest in reading spiritual literature	Expresses being abandoned by or having anger toward God
Poor coping	Expresses alienation		Inability to experience the transcendent
			Requests to see a religious leader
			Sudden changes in spiritual practices
			Inability to be introspective/ inward turning
			Expresses being without hope, suffering

Like the list of spiritual needs, the list of clinical signs of distress varies from one author to another, depending on the methodology used to identify them. Caregivers are encouraged to be aware of the signs of spiritual distress and to identify those shown by their patients.

---

13 NANDA International, "Détresse spirituelle": 439.

There is a practical consensus in the biomedical literature about the fact that a state of spiritual distress requires intervention. A comparison of the various definitions of need and distress reveals clearly that distress is considered as a pathological deviation from the norm that is more severe than the deviation of need, and often requires an intervention to correct the situation. Actual implementation will, of course, require consent from the patient, who will be able to choose the type of support and the person or persons who will provide it.[14]

5.1.1.2 Critique of the terms of need and distress

Although the terms "need" and "distress" are frequently used in research and clinical practice to describe the spiritual experience during illness, and although they appear to cause no particular difficulties for users on a daily basis, they still raise some questions in terms of epistemology because they are linked to knowledge of the spiritual experience.

My first remark concerns the distinction between need and desire. The underlying problem is the determination of the nature of the gap experienced between the actual spiritual state and the ideal state encapsulated in the biomedical definition of spirituality and its operational concept of spiritual wellbeing. How should this gap be named and qualified, from a spiritual point of view? But above all, how should the tension experienced by the subject be interpreted? If the gap is expressed in a clinical setting, should it immediately be considered a focus of care? We will attempt to answer these questions by exploring the distinction between need and desire.

Awareness of a gap between the state experienced *hic et nunc* and the "target" ideal is transposed psychologically and existentially into tension of various forms and various kinds, depending on its object.

In a test to shed more light on the need/desire distinction, Louis Roy reported a convergence between the approaches to the topic in various fields (theology, philosophy, psychoanalysis, psychology).[15] The following quote summarizes the situation well: "While a need is *something to be consumed*, desire is *someone*

---

14 Patients may have a choice between a person from their own religious or spiritual tradition, and a spiritual worker, if the service exists in the care institution. Depending on the country concerned, the spiritual workers recognized by care institutions may have a specific title: "aumô-nier" in France and Belgium, "accompagnant spirituel" in French-speaking Switzerland, "intervenant ou intervenante en soins spirituels" in Québec, "chaplain" in the English-speaking world, etc.

15 "Description du désir": Louis Roy, *Libérer le désir* (Montréal: Médiaspaul, 2009), 11–29.

with whom to communicate."[16] Unpacked, this statement means that a need is met by assimilating, or making our own, something "other" that is seen as an object,[17] while a desire is a feeling of being drawn to someone who will always remain "other", neither assimilable nor reducible to an object. Meeting a need destroys the object coveted and calms the need temporarily, until it is felt again. The need is met when the other is "assimilated", made one's own, and disappears as a result. In contrast, desire grows and is not extinguished, even if the communication is successful. The happy paradox of desire is to grow deeper and to never be met, even after contact with the desired being.

This distinction is not echoed in clinical culture, where it appears without purpose.[18] Like the distinction religion/spirituality that appears to be more suitable for theoretical debate than clinical application[19], the terms "need" and "desire" are, at best, used as synonyms.

Based on this exploration of the terms "need" and "desire", are clinicians and theoreticians engaged in a fruitless dialogue? Yes, if only the above positions are considered. However, it appears possible to uphold certain elements of each term, if the appropriate qualifications are made.

First, we must recognize that use of the expressions "spiritual need" and "spiritual distress" has a certain relevance. They make exchanges of information and a uniform use of language possible between caregivers. They open a window onto this aspect of the experience of illness; they make it clinically visible and understandable for caregivers. From this point of view, these two clinical concepts are heuristically useful and support a global consideration of what the patient is experiencing.

However, at the spiritual support stage, which is not primarily a clinical responsibility, chaplains must be able to distinguish between a need and a desire,

---

16 Roy, *Libérer le désir*, 13. [translation]. Roy cites theologian and philosopher Benoît Garceau.
17 Whatever the nature of the "other".
18 Dominique Jacquemin, ed. *Besoins spirituels. Soins, désir, responsabilités*, vol. 7, Soins et spiritualités (Bruxelles: Lumen vitae, 2016), 11–16. "La parole aux médecins" [translation]. In an interview reported in the book, one physician states: "I have never paid attention to the distinction between need and desire in connection with spirituality. I am happy to let theologians discuss it at length. In my practice, I regularly mix need and desire [...]. They are words that I am happy to use in place of each other in a spontaneous discussion or multi-professional conversations about a patient. From my point of view, in the field, the distinction is not useful." Jacquemin, *Besoins spirituels. Soins, désir, responsabilités*, 14.
19 Harold G. Koenig, "Religion, spirituality, and health: the research and clinical implications," *ISRN Psychiatry* (2012); Harold G. Koenig, Verna Benner Carson, and Dana E. King, *Handbook of religion and health*, 2nd ed. (Oxford: Oxford University Press, 2012), 48.

for a simple reason: spiritual life does not follow the logic of an "other" that can be consumed or assimilated, generating immediate satisfaction. Accompaniment for spiritual desire is provided as part of a dynamic that is not part of the dimension of survival, but is part of the question of meaning, the meaning of life taken as a whole, "a life of plenitude"[20] in the words of Pierre-Yves Brandt. Spiritual life is not limited to needs; it is a desire for plenitude that deepens with moments of often fleeting contact with the desired "object".

Besides this distinction between survival and a life of "plenitude", there is another reason for carefully taking the need/desire distinction into account in clinical practice. Describing a spiritual quest as part of the dynamic of desire protects against the temptation of offering clinical solutions to situations that, in fact, come under the heading of accompaniment. To succumb to this temptation would be to accept a form of medicalization of the spiritual state.

My second epistemological remark concerns the way in which the healthcare world "addresses" the spiritual experience through the concepts and notions it applies. As we saw above, the concepts that operationalize the concern for a patient's spiritual experience are interlinked: the notion of spiritual wellbeing positing an optimal spiritual state, and the notions of need and distress describing the gap between this theoretical optimal state and the patient's actual state. This conceptual system is built on the health/pathology dichotomy which, needless to say, is a central element in medical thought and clinical action. Just as a declaration that a physical or mental state is "pathological" leads to a care-oriented or medical intervention, so the identification of a need or distress in the spiritual realm encourages an action or gesture by the members of the care team, which may include a person providing spiritual accompaniment.

In contrast, the traditions of spiritual accompaniment in Western Christianity[21] distinguish two types of "asperity" in a personal spiritual progression: spiritual pathology[22] and spiritual crisis.[23] The expression "spiritual pathology" in the Christian tradition of spiritual accompaniment designates subjective experi-

---

20 Pierre-Yves Brandt, "La spiritualité: réponse à un besoin, à une soif ou à une quête?," in *Besoins spirituels: soins, désir, responsabilités*, ed. Eckhard Frick, Dominique Jacquemin, and Cosette Odier (Bruxelles: Lumen vitae, 2016): 31.

21 It is important to introduce here, only too quickly, the difference on this point between Western and Eastern Christianity. Eastern Christianity developed an ascetic tradition that became a genuine diagnostic and therapeutic method for spiritual illnesses.

22 Gian-F. Zuanazzi, "Pathologie spirituelle," in *Dictionnaire de la vie spirituelle*, ed. Stefano De Fiores and Tullo Goffi (Paris: Cerf, 1983).

23 L. De Candido, "Crise," in *Dictionnaire de la vie spirituelle*, ed. Stefano De Fiores and Tullo Goffi (Paris: Cerf, 1983).

ences of "unjustified guilt or, on the contrary, [the impossibility] of making a moral judgment" [24] and, in addition, scruples and delirium.[25] A spiritual crisis is considered to be a crucial moment, a choice "[a] decisive moment, [a] determining threshold, [a] turning point in a situation."[26] Although it may take one of several forms of self-questioning,[27] it is primarily understood as a tipping point between two forms of integration of spiritual life or a moment of transition between two phases of "development" of spiritual life.[28] In short, a crisis can be seen as part of a progression or coherent life story, even if it is experienced as something difficult or negative by the person concerned. A person in crisis may need accompaniment at this time, but this is not necessarily "treatment", because the crisis is not pathological in itself.[29]

5.1.2 Tools

The development of tools to support a clinical judgment is part of the research tradition in the field of biomedicine. Whether the goal is to detect or assess a pa-

---

24 Zuanazzi, "Pathologie spirituelle," 803.
25 Zuanazzi, "Pathologie spirituelle," 807.
26 De Candido, "Crise," 218.
27 De Candido identifies three main types of spiritual crisis: a theologal crisis concerning the relationship with God, an ethical crisis concerning the relationship with oneself and others, and the institutional crisis which, as its names indicates, concerns the key institutions of religious life: family, Church, sacraments, priesthood, consecrated religious life, vocation. De Candido, "Crise," 225–28.
28 Fritz Oser and Paul Gmünder, *L'homme, son développement religieux. Étude de structuralisme génétique*, trans. Louis Ridez, Sciences humaines et religions (Paris: Cerf, 1991[1988]). I have put quotation marks around "development" to highlight the fact that this bibliographical reference is part of a common approach in the 20ᵗʰ century inspired by the work of Jean Piaget. However, here, it does not matter whether or not the approach is modern, since spiritual maturation has always been, and still is, seen as a progression by Christianity.
29 The idea of spiritual illness exists in the Christian spiritual traditions, whether in Catholic theology: Adolphe Tanquerey, *Précis de théologie ascétique et mystique*, 8e ed. (Paris: Desclée, 1923). Or, above all, in Orthodox tradition: Jean-Claude Larchet, *Thérapeutique des maladies spirituelles*, 2 vols., vol. 1, l'Arbre de Jessé (Paris: Éditions de l'Ancre, 1991). In other cases, the notions of spiritual illness and remedy are used in the same way, as "medical images", or as striking symbols that seek to recognize the effect of sin on the human soul (Larchet, *Thérapeutique des maladies spirituelles*, 1, 9.) The "medical image" is first and foremost a borrowing from medical language by theology, for strictly pastoral purposes. It is important to avoid the mistake to using the medical vocabulary to designate the spiritual experience during illness, which is not a theological category. Readers can see chapter 3 for a discussion of the analogy between health and salvation.

tient's state, diagnosis, the determination of suitable treatment, intervention, and the provision of information for patients and their families, tools exist for addressing situations using procedures or templates for action of varying degrees of complexity, validated on the basis of the theoretical and practical standards in force.[30] This "tool-based" approach to illness and therapy is also seen in the way in which the clinical world addresses the spiritual experience of the sick.

The tools used for the spiritual experience during illness correspond to three main steps which match, more or less, the steps in a clinical judgment. These steps are: spiritual anamnesis, spiritual evaluation and spiritual intervention. It goes without saying that these "protocolized" ways of approaching the spiritual experience are not part of the religious traditions, except for anamnesis and spiritual evaluation.

5.1.2.1 Spiritual anamnesis

Spiritual anamnesis is a search for information about a patient's spiritual and religious background. The tools developed for this purpose allow professional caregivers to find out more about the patient's history and religious or spiritual views. As in the anamnesis of systems (cardiovascular, respiratory, etc.), the professional asks open-ended questions to gather information and better understand the current situation by comparing it to the patient's antecedents. The information collected during a spiritual anamnesis is not an intervention in the strict meaning of the term, since it does not require advanced knowledge or special skills in theology, religion or spiritual accompaniment. Anamnesis may be practised by a care professional with a minimum of training. The literature provides ethical guidelines that define the involvement of care professionals in the gathering of information: make referrals to chaplains, spiritual directors, or community resources as appropriate; respect a patient's privacy; do not impose one's beliefs on others; do not make value judgments about beliefs and practices, etc.[31]

The tools for spiritual anamnesis proposed in the biomedical literature have a similar structure, with several typical stages.[32] Using the HOPE questionnaire as an example, we can see what the main stages in anamnesis are.

---

30 A classic example is the FACIT (Functional Assessment of Chronic Illness Therapy) system, based on HRQOL (Health Related Quality of Life) measurements.
31 Christina M. Puchalski and Anna L. Romer, "Taking a Spiritual History Allows Clinicians to Understand Patients More Fully," *Journal of Palliative Medicine* 3, no. 1 (2000).
32 Eckhard Frick et al., "A clinical interview assessing cancer patients' spiritual needs and preferences," *European Journal of Cancer Care* 15, no. 3 (2006); Gowri Anandarajah and Ellen Hight, "Spirituality and medical practice: using the HOPE questions as a practical tool for spiritual as-

Table 4. Examples of Questions for the HOPE Approach to Spiritual Assessment[33]

H:

Sources of hope, meaning, comfort, strength, peace, love and connection

- We have been discussing your support systems. I was wondering, what is there in your life that gives you internal support?
- What are your sources of hope, strength, comfort and peace?
- What do you hold on to during difficult times?
- What sustains you and keeps you going?
- For some people, their religious or spiritual beliefs act as a source of comfort and strength in dealing with life's ups and downs; is this true for you?

If the answer is "Yes," go on to O and P questions.

If the answer is "No," consider asking: Was it ever? If the answer is "Yes," ask: What changed?

O:

Organized religion

- Do you consider yourself part of an organized religion?
- How important is this to you?
- What aspects of your religion are helpful and not so helpful to you?
- Are you part of a religious or spiritual community? Does it help you? How?

P:

Personal spirituality/ practices

- Do you have personal spiritual beliefs that are independent of organized religion? What are they?
- Do you believe in God? What kind of relationship do you have with God?
- What aspects of your spirituality or spiritual practices do you find most helpful to you personally? (e. g., prayer, meditation, reading scripture, attending religious services, listening to music, hiking, communing with nature)

E:

Effects on medical care and end-of-life issues

- Has being sick (or your current situation) affected your ability to do the things that usually help you spiritually? (Or affected your relationship with God?)
- As a doctor, is there anything that I can do to help you access the resources that usually help you?
- Are you worried about any conflicts between your beliefs and your medical situation/care/ decisions?
- Would it be helpful for you to speak to a clinical chaplain/community spiritual leader?

---

sessment," *American Family Physician* 63, no. 1 (2001); Puchalski and Romer, "Taking a Spiritual History Allows Clinicians to Understand Patients More Fully"; Christina M. Puchalski, "The FICA Spiritual History Tool #274," *J Palliat Med* 17, no. 1 (2014).

33 Anandarajah and Hight, "Spirituality and medical practice: using the HOPE questions as a practical tool for spiritual assessment".

Table 4. Examples of Questions for the HOPE Approach to Spiritual Assessment *(continued)*

- Are there any specific practices or restrictions I should know about in providing your medical care? (e. g., dietary restrictions, use of blood products)
- If the patient is dying: How do your beliefs affect the kind of medical care you would like me to provide over the next few days/weeks/months?

The first stage (H) addresses the place of spirituality or religion in the person's everyday life. The goal is to establish if it provides support at difficult times, such as illness. The second stage (O) verifies membership of a religious denomination or community of religious practice. These questions show that it cannot be assumed that a person belongs to a particular group, even after stating in the first stage that religion or spirituality are important. In secularized societies, membership in an organized religion takes many forms, from fervent adherents who observe the doctrine strictly, to modes in which believers may hold opinions that diverge from the doctrine of the group. In short, religious membership is complex phenomenon, and this must be taken into account when interpreting the data gathered through anamnesis.

The third stage (P) focuses on individual practices, and is also important if the individuality and uniqueness of the sick person is to be respected. People can adopt the religious or spiritual practices that are most suitable for them, meaning that they may diverge from the official beliefs of the group. For example, in Québec, it is not unusual to meet Christians who believe in reincarnation even though, from the standpoint of Christian doctrine, it is a belief that contradicts the very essence of Christianity. The question here is not to judge the compliance of the patient's beliefs with those of the religious group concerned, but to note the singularity of the patient's story and beliefs. The sensitivity of care professionals to this individual profile will prevent over-hasty judgements and the imposition of rites and belief systems.[34] The other important aspect of this stage is the identification of the practices already applied by the person during the episode of illness. The precious clues provided by the patient will help draw up a better overview of his or her story and spiritual or religious background, and will also help caregivers plan their clinical actions while being careful to respect, as far as possible, the times that are important for the patient, which requires a careful balancing of care times and times of religious or spiritual recovery.

---

[34] I once met a Catholic priest who anointed all the patients he met, since everyone in his region was baptized and Catholic. This is the type of unsupported generalization that does not take the uniqueness of individual pathways into account.

The last stage (E) is when the types of activities and spiritual interventions that may be reasonably organized during the care episode are planned. This may range from defining a prescribed menu (in order to respect food-related rules connected with a religious belief or lifestyle) to organizing change of location to allow participation in liturgical events within the institution; or organizing the room layout, planning visits by representatives of the religious or spiritual community, organizing meetings with in-house staff providing spiritual accompaniment, and so on. Respect for the commitments made at this stage demonstrates the sincerity of the care team's interest in the patient's spiritual life.

As we can see, anamnesis leads to several results. The first is the gathering of information on the person's current spiritual life, which is not limited to the spiritual experience during the time of illness. The second is the opportunity to record some of the patient's spiritual history, depending on the openness of the patient and the perspicacity of the care professional conducting the interview. This spiritual history could add perspective to the results of a spiritual evaluation. Last, anamnesis contributes to a consolidation of the bond of trust between the patient and the care team.

5.1.2.2 Spiritual evaluation

The objective of spiritual evaluation is to determine the current state of a patient presenting the signs associated with spiritual distress,[35] whatever the care sector.[36] The evaluation ascertains whether or not the patient is experiencing spiri-

---

35 See the previous section.

36 Harvey Max Chochinov et al., "The patient dignity inventory: a novel way of measuring dignity-related distress in palliative care," *J Pain Symptom Manage* 36, no. 6 (2008); Sian Cotton et al., "Spirituality and religion in patients with HIV/AIDS," *J Gen Intern Med* 21 Suppl 5 (2006); Sabine Fischbeck et al., "Assessing somatic, psychosocial, and spiritual distress of patients with advanced cancer: development of the Advanced Cancer Patients' Distress Scale," *Am J Hosp Palliat Care* 30, no. 4 (2013); Sachiko Gomi, Vincent R. Starnino, and Edward R. Canda, "Spiritual assessment in mental health recovery," *Community Mental Health Journal* 50, no. 4 (2014); Sylvia Mohr et al., "The assessment of spirituality and religiousness in schizophrenia," *Journal of Nervous and Mental Disease*, no. 195 (2007); Stéfanie Monod-Zorzi et al., "Validation of the Spiritual Distress Assessment Tool in older hospitalized patients," *BMC Geriatr* 12 (2012); Stéfanie M. Monod et al., "The spiritual distress assessment tool: an instrument to assess spiritual distress in hospitalised elderly persons," *BMC Geriatr* 10 (2010); Cassandra Vieten et al., "Spiritual and religious competencies for psychologists," *Psychology of Religion and Spirituality* 5, no. 3 (2013); Faye Weinstein et al., "Spirituality Assessments and Interventions in Pain Medicine." Vertical Health LLC, http://www.practicalpainmanagement.com/treatments/psychological/spirituality-assessments-interventions-pain-medicine.

tual distress.[37] Two types of tools have been developed over the years: question-naires—presented as a "measurement" tool—and the tools used during a discussion with the patient. In other words, evaluation tools are either quantitative or dialogue-based, with the quantitative tools being more numerous and more commonly applied.

Table 5. Daily Spiritual Experience Scale[38]

	Many Times a Day	Everyday	Most Days	Some Days	Once in a While	Never or Almost Never
I feel God's presence	1	2	3	4	5	6
I experience a connection all life	1	2	3	4	5	6
During worship, or at other times when connecting with God, I feel joy, which lifts me out of my daily concerns.	1	2	3	4	5	6
I find strength in my religion or spirituality	1	2	3	4	5	6
I find comfort in my religion or spirituality	1	2	3	4	5	6
I feel deep inner peace or harmony	1	2	3	4	5	6
I ask for God's help in the midst of daily activities	1	2	3	4	5	6
I feel God's love for me directly	1	2	3	4	5	6
I fell God's love for me through others	1	2	3	4	5	6

---

37 The categories of anamnesis and spiritual assessment are sometimes confused in the biomedical literature. In some cases, the anamnesis step is included in assessment: Tami Borneman, Betty Ferrell, and Christina M. Puchalski, "Evaluation of the FICA Tool for Spiritual Assessment," *J Pain Symptom Manage* 40, no. 2 (2010). This telescoping of categories ignores the different goals of each stage—for anamnesis, gathering information on the patient's history and spiritual life and, as we will see, a determination of the patient's current state. Anamnesis takes a broad view of spiritual experience, including the past and the patient's spiritual life prior to the illness, whereas an assessment looks only at the patient's current state. The difference can be expressed as an analogy: assessment is to anamnesis as a snapshot is to a feature film.
38 Lynn G. Underwood and Jeanne A. Teresi, "The daily spiritual experience scale: development, theoretical description, reliability, exploratory factor analysis, and preliminary construct validity using health-related data," *Ann Behav Med* 24, no. 1 (2002).

Table 5. Daily Spiritual Experience Scale *(continued)*

	Many Times a Day	Everyday	Most Days	Some Days	Once in a While	Never or Almost Never
I am spiritually touched by the beauty of creation	1	2	3	4	5	6
I feel thankful for my blessings	1	2	3	4	5	6
I feel a selfless caring for others	1	2	3	4	5	6
I accept others even when they do things that I think are wrong	1	2	3	4	5	6
I desire to be closer to God or in union with Him	1	2	3	4	5	6

	Not Close at All	Somewhat Close	Very Close	As Close as Possible
In general, how close do you feel to God?	1	2	3	4

The quantitative tools vary,[39] but share a basic outline. They are made up of series of statements of a spiritual nature (see the example), most of which point to an ideal spiritual state, generally derived from the definitions of spirituality and spiritual wellbeing developed as part of the biomedical discourse[40]: "I feel at peace", "I can find within myself the resources I need to face illness", "I have a reason for living", etc. For each statement, the patient indicates his or her

---

39 FACIT-Sp in Amy H. Peterman et al., "Measuring spiritual well-being in people with cancer: the functional assessment of chronic illness therapy–Spiritual Well-being Scale (FACIT-Sp)," *Ann Behav Med* 24, no. 1 (2002); Amy H. Peterman et al., "Measuring meaning and peace with the FACIT-spiritual well-being scale: distinction without a difference?," *Psychol Assess* 26, no. 1 (2014). The Spirituality Index of Well-Being in Timothy P. Daaleman and Bruce B. Frey, "The Spirituality Index of Well-Being: a new instrument for health-related quality-of-life research," *Annals Of Family Medicine* 2, no. 5 (2004). The Brief Serenity Scale in Mary Jo Kreitzer et al., "The Brief Serenity Scale: A Psychometric Analysis of a Measure of Spirituality and Well-Being," *Journal of Holistic Nursing* 27, no. 1 (2009). The Daily Spiritual Experience Scale Underwood and Teresi, "The daily spiritual experience scale: development, theoretical description, reliability, exploratory factor analysis, and preliminary construct validity using health-related data".
40 Nicolas Vonarx and Mireille Lavoie, "Soins infirmiers et spiritualité: d'une démarche systématique à l'accueil d'une expérience," *Revue internationale de soins palliatifs* 26, no. 4 (2011).

agreement using a Likert scale. By adding up the numerical value of each answer, a score is calculated that represents the patient's state at the time of completing the questionnaire. For the tools containing a majority of statements that reflect an ideal state, the lower the score, the more likelihood that the patient is in some form of "spiritual distress".

The final score generated by a quantitative tool is not, and cannot be used as, a diagnosis. A judgment concerning a patient's spiritual state cannot rely solely on the score generated by a spiritual evaluation tool. The score indicates the person's state and may be included in a more holistic judgement that takes other factors and data into account, such as the information collected during spiritual anamnesis.

Dialogue-based tools are completely different. They comprise a grid of key points that must be covered in a conversation, during which the person providing spiritual accompaniment identifies the clues that will be used to make a judgment about the person's state. A clear example is the STIV model produced by an interdisciplinary team at the university hospital centre for the French-speaking canton of Vaud in Switzerland.[41]

Table 6. Presentation of the STIV

Sub-dimension	Definition of the sub-dimension	Need	Example of question	Example of need not covered
Meaning	What gives life a direction and sense and allows an overall life balance to be maintained	Overall life balance	Are you having difficulty experiencing/coping with what is happening (illness/hospitalization, etc.)?	"I know I must cope with it, and find a new balance, but I can't … I don't have the strength"
Transcendence	Foundation located outside the individual that provides grounding, relationship with the ultimate, element(s) that go	Connection with transcendence	Has what is happening to you changed your relationship with God (closer, more distant, the same)?	"… I think that God has abandoned me …" "I can't paint anymore, and painting was the only think that connected me

---

41 Monod-Zorzi et al., "Validation of the Spiritual Distress Assessment Tool in older hospitalized patients"; Monod et al., "The spiritual distress assessment tool: an instrument to assess spiritual distress in hospitalised elderly persons"; Stéfanie Monod-Zorzi, *Soins aux personnes âgées. Intégrer la spiritualité?*, ed. Eckhard Frick and Cosette Odier, vol. 2, Soins et spiritualités (Bruxelles: Lumen vitae, 2012).

Table 6. Presentation of the STIV *(continued)*

Sub-dimension	Definition of the sub-dimension	Need	Example of question	Example of need not covered
	beyond the individual and are used by the individual to name his or her existential dependency			to the force that helped me advance ..."
Values	Value system that determines what is good and true for the individual. The system is made apparent by the individual's actions and choices.	Value 1: Need for caregivers to understand what has value for me	Do you think that the people caring for you know enough about your life history?	"... I am just a number here ... nobody knows who I really am ..."
Psycho-social identity	The patient's environment, including society, caregivers, family members and friends, together help maintain the individual's unique identity.	Need to maintain one's identity	Do you suffer from solitude? Can you give me an image of yourself in your current situation?	"My friends don't come to see me ... My family doesn't understand what I am going through ... I no longer recognize myself ..."

The grid is used to evaluate spiritual needs, and is applied during a conversation between the chaplain and the sick person, whether hospitalized or not. It helps the chaplain direct the discussion, following which he or she will be able to qualify the patient's state for each of the four sub-dimensions and make a judgment about the patient's overall state.

5.1.2.3 Overview of evaluation tools

The use of spiritual evaluation tools in clinical practice has both strengths and weaknesses.

The strengths include that they can be used by professionals, after receiving sufficient training. Although both types of tools produce results that must be refocused and analyzed, it remains true that quantitative tools are easier to work with than dialogue-based tools, which require training in spiritual accompaniment if they are to be fully effective in identifying the patient's state.

Next, the tools make it possible to describe, in clinical terms, religious and spiritual experiences that are harder to identify using traditional terminology. For example, the reality named as "spiritual distress" is easier to understand than if it was designated by the traditional expression "purgative way" used in ascetical and mystical theology, or the expression "night of the senses" often used by mystics to designate a period of "spiritual drought".

Last, the tools, "translate" religious and spiritual experiences into a language that the members of an interdisciplinary care team can understand, easing the flow of information between the team members.

However, the evaluation tools also have some weaknesses.

First, as mentioned above, their content is based on a restrictive conception of the spiritual experience during illness. By giving priority to wellbeing and harmony as indicators of spiritual health, they may exclude legitimate spiritual experiences that fail to comply with the biomedical definition of spirituality[42] such as, for example, a patient's anger at imminent death combined with a feeling that they are abandoning the people they are leaving behind, or incomprehension when faced with the absurdity of suffering and illness. In light of the points raised above, the reduction of the spiritual experience to wellbeing and harmony leads to a form of standardization and even to the pathologization of anything that falls outside the framework of the biomedical interpretation. In short, restricting the ideal spiritual experience to wellbeing and harmony may lead to its medicalization. This possible practical repercussion arises from the application of the health/pathology paradigm, as used in healthcare, to the spiritual experience during illness. Not only may certain experiences be excluded, but any spiritual experience with negative connotations according to the tool used may be wrongly interpreted. To make an analogy with diagnostic tests, the tools may create "false positives" by identifying spiritual distress where none exists.[43] The mere possibility of creating "false positives", inherent in any form of evaluation, explains the need for prudence highlighted above and for placing the results of a spiritual evaluation in a clinical context in the long-term perspective of the sick person's religious and spiritual history.

I will make one final remark in conclusion to this presentation of tools for spiritual evaluation, concerning the link between anamnesis and spiritual evaluation. A spiritual evaluation provides an instantaneous portrait which, even though it describes the present state, must be set against a life journey. By placing an instant portrait of the person's spiritual state against the background of

---

42 Jobin, "Êtes-vous en belle santé? Sur l'esthétisation de la spiritualité en biomédecine".
43 A false positive results from a procedure or test that indicates a problem where none exists.

the person's spiritual history, provided the care team has access to it and the conditions needed to manage it, the evaluation results will be seen in their true light. In other words, a spiritual evaluation based on the categories of need and distress cannot dispense with a religious or spiritual anamnesis, in the form of an elucidation of the patient's religious and spiritual journey and beliefs. In more technical terms, the issue of a language of diagnosis based on the categories of need and distress is an issue of temporality. More specifically, it involves the gap between the instantaneous nature of the diagnosis, compared to the duration (however variable) of a life. Before defining the severity of a spiritual state, there must be an opportunity to compare the "deviation" with the sick person's habitual state.

It is fair to object that it is not always possible to place the current diagnosis on a longer temporal timeframe. In an emergency, or if the sick person is unwilling to share, a spiritual anamnesis cannot always be completed. These technical difficulties, however, do not invalidate the underlying principle, which is that the interpretation of a specific moment in a person's life is only credible is it is placed against the context of the person's life journey.[44] The spiritual state at a given point in time cannot be separated from the spiritual identity deployed and consolidated over a much larger timespan. In fact, this is the reason why, in religious traditions, spiritual accompaniment is always conceived of and carried out in a relationship that covers a period of months and even years. Once again, although spiritual accompaniment during a period of illness takes place over a shorter time, the guiding principle that a spiritual state should be interpreted against the background of a lifelong journey or referred to a spiritual identity requires a prudent use (however achieved) of the results of a spiritual evaluation.

5.1.2.4 Spiritual intervention

The third type of tool is associated with spiritual intervention, in other words any form of action taken to accompany a patient in a specific spiritual or religious process. Support, prayer, rites, the reading of sacred texts, silent presence, ther-

---

44 The bibliography on the connection between personal identity and life story is extensive. In this field, the work of Paul Ricoeur, on the one hand, and of narratologists working in healthcare, on the other, are the main authorities. Cf. Paul Ricoeur, *Soi-même comme un autre*, Points essais, 330 (Paris: Seuil, 1990); Rita Charon, *Narrative medicine: honoring the stories of illness* (New York: Oxford University Press, 2008); Arthur W. Frank, *The Wounded Storyteller. Body, Illness, and Ethics* (Chicago: The University of Chicago Press, 1995); Arthur W. Frank, *Letting stories breathe: a socio-narratology* (Chicago: University of Chicago Press, 2010).

apeutic touch, support groups, etc., are all actions that may be considered to be forms of spiritual intervention. They may derive from a particular religious or spiritual tradition, or may be created *ad hoc*. Intervention does not require a prior evaluation—a rite may be implemented even if there is no need to address or distress to "care for". Spiritual intervention may occur at the request of the patient or the patient's family, whether to comfort the patient or for other reasons: to celebrate a person's life at its end; to transmit a symbolic heritage to those left behind; to celebrate a recovery or improving health; to find new energy to persevere with difficult treatments; etc.

Various codified forms of spiritual intervention are often encountered. The western religious and spiritual traditions are replete with rites (private and public) for times of sickness or imminent death.[45] The *Ars moriendi* tradition, a series of spiritual exercises in contemplation of death, can be traced back to the 15th century, and was intended to "ensure salvation for one's soul and avoid a second death, the most terrifying for a believer since it involves damnation."[46] Through prayers, times of introspection and rites, the *Ars moriendi* offered a time of preparation and, if needed, purification. The influence of *Ars moriendi* led to other traditions, including the *Exhortations aux mourants*[47] and the literary genre of "preparation for death", one of the most famous of which was written and published by the humanist Erasmus at the end of his life.[48] By providing a structure[49] for the hours leading up to death and a practical guide to accompaniment[50] the *Ars moriendi* was a educational tool.[51] Behind these preparations for death lay the ideal of a good death or, at least, a death in the proper conditions.

"Protocolized" accompaniment at the end of a person's life is now accomplished using means other than the traditional *Ars moriendi*. However, the idea of accompanying death using a process that includes themes and has a de-

---

45 Everyday life can also provide a setting for "protocolized" support even in the absence of illness or impending death. One example is the spiritual tradition initiated by Ignatius of Loyola, the founder of the Jesuits, which includes spiritual exercises for everyday life, a four-step process for deepening one's spiritual identity and relationship with God.

46 Bayard, *L'art de bien mourir au XVe siècle*, 14.

47 "Ars moriendi," in *Dictionnaire de spiritualité ascétique et mystique*, ed. Marcel Viller (Paris: Beauchesne, 1935).

48 *Érasme, La préparation à la mort*.

49 Bayard, *L'art de bien mourir au XVe siècle*, 77–104.

50 Bayard, *L'art de bien mourir au XVe siècle*, 107–42.

51 This paragraph is taken from Jacques Cherblanc and Guy Jobin, "Vers une psychologisation du religieux ? Le cas des institutions sanitaires au Québec," *Archives de sciences sociales des religions* 163, no. 3 (2013).

gree of "therapeutic" content remains. Dignity therapy, proposed by Canadian psychiatrist Harvey M. Chochinov[52] seeks to appease the existential distress that may occur at the end of a person's life[53] and which is behind many requests for euthanasia or medically-assisted suicide.[54]

Last, the current fascination with mindfulness, or "the art of facing difficulties, leading to effective solutions, inner peace and harmony,"[55] should be mentioned in connection with the move towards the protocolization of spiritual accompaniment. Mindfulness combats stress, seen as a pathology that can be "cured", by "establishing a new relationship with illness, incapacity, and even death, to the extent that we learn to see it holistically."[56]

5.1.2.5 Who is responsible for spiritual intervention?

Who can provide spiritual accompaniment in the healthcare world? The question is not redundant—in addition to the people with training and due accreditation who provide spiritual accompaniment, several care professions have claimed an interest and competency in providing spiritual accompaniment. Many reasons are given for these claims, depending on the profession concerned. They range from historical, identity-based arguments (nursing and social work are both professions that emerged in the 19th century in a religious environment), to arguments based on the holistic nature of care that must consider a sick person as a whole (here again, we find nursing and social work, as well as occupational therapy, clinical psychology and other professions). Last, it is important not to underestimate the role played by volunteers providing spiritual accompani-

---

52 Harvey Max Chochinov, "Dignity Therapy: A Novel Psychotherapeutic Intervention for Patients near the End of Life," *Journal of Clinical Oncology* 23, no. 4 (2005); Harvey Max Chochinov, "Dying, Dignity, and New Horizons in Palliative End-of-Life Care," *CA A Cancer Journal for the Clinicians* 56 (2006); Harvey Max Chochinov, "Dignity and the essence of medicine: the A, B, C, and D of dignity conserving care," *Bmj* 335, no. 7612 (2007); Harvey Max Chochinov, "Dignity-Based Approaches in the Care of Terminally Ill Patients," *Current Opinion in Supportive and Palliative Care* 2 (2008); Harvey Max Chochinov et al., "Effect of dignity therapy on distress and end-of-life experience in terminally ill patients: a randomised controlled trial," *Lancet Oncol* 12, no. 8 (2011).
53 Pierre Gagnon et al., "Le rôle central des questions existentielles et spirituelles en oncologie et en soins palliatifs," in *Spiritualités et biomédecine Enjeux d'une intégration*, ed. Guy Jobin, Jean-Marc Charron, and Michel Nyabenda (Québec: Presses de l'Université Laval, 2013).
54 Chochinov, "Dignity Therapy: A Novel Psychotherapeutic Intervention for Patients near the End of Life".
55 Jon Kabat-Zinn, *Au coeur de la tourmente, la pleine conscience*, ed. Ahmed Djouder, Bien-être (Paris: Éditions J'ai lu, 2009[1990]).
56 Kabat-Zinn, *Au coeur de la tourmente, la pleine conscience*, 313.

ment,[57] who see it as a way to demonstrate their commitment to and solidarity with the sick.

This question raises a complex problem with a range of factors that will be used to determine who is authorized by the healthcare institution to provide spiritual accompaniment on its premises. The first factor is the system in place in a given country to regulate religious matters, which is then transposed into specific arrangements within the institution. For example, in France, in public institutions which are officially non-denominational, spiritual accompaniment is generally provided under contract by outside players grouped together in a multi-denominational chaplaincy. As a result, representatives from various religious communities and groups are given a mandate to accompany the sick. On the other hand, there are also groups of lay volunteers who offer spiritual accompaniment in the home. In Québec, where public healthcare institutions are also officially non-denominational, the law and the departmental guidelines on health and social services stipulate that institutions must provide "safe, continuous and accessible quality health or social services which respect the rights and spiritual needs of individuals."[58] This obligation is met by the institution by setting up a non-denominational service for spiritual care. Given that no model is specified by law, it is up to the management of each institution to configure its service on the basis of the resources available.

In fact, the question is closely linked to the notion of professionalism[59] in the healthcare world and the ethical question of the skills needed to provide spiritual accompaniment.

---

57 For Québec, see: Gilles Nadeau, "Le coeur s'agrandit," in *Le bénévolat en soins palliatifs ou l'art d'accompagner*, ed. Andrée Sévigny, Manon Champagne, and Manal Guirguis-Younger (Québec: Maison Michel-Sarrazin/Presses de l'Université Laval, 2013); Guy Jobin et al., "Bénévolat et spiritualité en soins palliatifs," in *Le bénévolat en soins palliatifs ou l'art d'accompagner*, ed. Andrée Sévigny, Manon Champagne, and Manal Guirguis-Younger (Québec: Maison Michel Sarrazin/Presses de l'Université Laval, 2013). For France: Châtel, "Les nouvelles cultures de l'accompagnement: les soins palliatifs, une voie 'spirituelle' dans une société de performance."; Tanguy Châtel, *Vivants jusqu'à la mort. Accompagner la souffrance spirituelle en fin de vie* (Paris: Albin Michel, 2013).

58 "Loi sur les services de santé et les services sociaux," in *S-42*, ed. Ministère de la santé et des services sociaux (Québec: Gouvernement du Québec, 2005), section 100.

59 Based on Georges A. Legault, we can define the terms "professionals" and "professionalization". Professionals provide a service to the community by intervening with individuals and institutions; and act on the basis of theoretical knowledge and practical expertise in the analysis of the problems facing the individuals and institutions that consult them. They have practical skills and theoretical knowledge with respect to actions, and are aware of the legal/professional/moral/ethical rules governing the exercise of the profession. Last, professionals reflect on their practice in all its dimensions: knowledge, skills and attitudes. Georges-A. Legault, *Profes-*

A strong trend became apparent during the 20th century in the field of spiritual accompaniment during times of illness: professionalization. This is not surprising, since accompaniment has evolved in the technoscientific and bureaucratic healthcare environment and has sought a credible and relevant way to make spiritual intervention part of the work of institutions that are home to healthcare professionals. In short, the trend towards professionalism is driven both by the requirements of the healthcare setting and by the goal of spiritual accompaniers to be taken seriously by the institution and, even more directly, by the interdisciplinary care teams. This process is supported by specific training programs across most of Western society, generally at the university level, by a growing quantity of specialized literature, and by practical research using the strictest qualitative and quantitative research standards.

However, this move towards the professionalization of spiritual accompaniment in the healthcare world has occurred just as other professionals have begun to claim the skills and know-how used to provide patients with spiritual accompaniment, as noted above.

Given this competitive aspect, how can we answer the crucial question, "Who provides accompaniment?"

To my mind the main issue is one of professional ethics, since it involves looking at the very nature of the professional action concerned. Two arguments guide this view. First, a professional is a person who acts not simply through good intentions, because unfortunately even a benevolent action can harm a vulnerable and fragile person. A professional is a person whose actions are determined by objective standards, supported by a body of knowledge validated by the research and practice community. A professional action is therefore an action that complies with rules and standards, and that can be reported using reasonable criteria. From this point of view, professional training has a clear ethical dimension, since it provides a framework for good intentions. Second, spiritual accompaniment requires specific skills at all times, and this is especially true during times of illness, when the patient is vulnerable and fragile. The person providing spiritual accompaniment must find an approach that avoids both proselytism and indifference. Knowledge of religious and spiritual traditions; skills in helping relationships; familiarity with a life of faith or spiritual life and their psychological drivers; the ability to determine whether or not to intervene in a situation where religious and spiritual beliefs are at stake; knowing when one

---

sionnalisme et délibération éthique (Québec: Presses de l'Université du Québec, 2007), 16. Professionalization is the "creation of new jobs in the service sector [that] sometimes require the integration of practical knowledge [and that] require the acquisition of theoretical knowledge specific to the discipline." (Legault, *Professionnalisme et délibération éthique*, 12.)

has reached one's own limits and when to call on outside resources; these are just some of the skills needed to provide spiritual accompaniment during times of illness.

These arguments based on professional ethics lead me to the conclusion that the professional in the best position to provide spiritual accompaniment is a person with suitable training whose skills have been recognized following a course of study equivalent to that followed by the other professionals with whom the person will collaborate in a work setting.

Nevertheless, it is clear that patients will in fact decide who to confide in with respect to their spiritual experience. In this area, respect for a patient's autonomy is a founding principle, to which we must add freedom of religion and religious freedom, especially when the patient is vulnerable and fragile. For this reason, the professional reflex is to ensure, first, that one does not exceed the limits of one's own skills and, second, that the patient is referred to an accompanier or person chosen by the patient.

By making the spiritual experience a potential focus of care, the biomedical world has drawn it into a new and unfamiliar epistemological and clinical framework. It has made the spiritual experience a field of practice and research in which a degree of medical power is exercised.

This is the first path for the sapientialization of spiritual life. We will now turn to the second path laid out by biomedicine.

5.2 The spiritual experience as a care adjuvant

This second, pragmatic approach sees the spiritual experience as a factor that can help achieve care objectives. In other words, the biomedical world believes that the spiritual experience can be used as a resource in the fields of curative medicine, chronic care and palliative care. In whatever way, the mobilization of the spiritual experience in clinical processes could influence the state of the patient's health (or ill-health). I have already briefly discussed the promotion of mindfulness as a factor for "healing" or, at least, stress reduction.[60] Something that appears self-evident in the case of psychological "disorders" may also apply to somatic medicine. Two examples, drawn respectively from the fields of nephrology and pain medicine, are given here.

---

60 *Kabat-Zinn, Au coeur de la tourmente, la pleine conscience.*

5.2.1 Spirituality in the field of nephrology[61]

The main issue in research into spirituality in the field of renal disease and treatment involves the crucial aspect of survival[62] and, more specifically, the contribution made by spirituality to the willingness of patients suffering from end-stage renal disease (ESRD) to adjust to and continue their treatment.[63]

One of the factors contributing to perseverance is the perception that patients have of the quality of their own lives. Kimmel et al.[64] have shown that patients' perception of their own quality of life depended more on psychosocial or spiritual factors than on the physical aspects of care, and this is confirmed by other studies.[65] Kimmel et al. state that "the implication of these findings is that if nephrologists want to provide comprehensive care and improve hemodialysis patients' quality of life, they need to pay more attention to their patients' physical symptoms and psychosocial and spiritual concerns."[66] This influence has been explored in various ways, even though current knowledge is still incomplete.[67]

For greater clarity, we will summarize the direction taken in this research as follows.

---

61 This part of the chapter is taken from a text prepared as part of an unpublished article. I thank Jacinthe Beauchamp, Denis Belliveau and Amanda Horsman for their cooperation.

62 Joann Spinale et al., "Spirituality, social support, and survival in hemodialysis patients," *Clinical Journal of the American Society of Nephrology* 3, no. 6 (2008).

63 Ruth A. Tanyi and Joan S. Werner, "Adjustment, spirituality, and health in women on hemodialysis," *Clinical Nursing Research* 12, no. 3 (2003); Joni Walton, "Finding a balance: a grounded theory study of spirituality in hemodialysis patients," *Nephrology Nursing Journal* 29, no. 5 (2002).

64 Paul L. Kimmel et al., "ESRD patient quality of life: symptoms, spiritual beliefs, psychosocial factors, and ethnicity," *American Journal of Kidney Diseases* 42, no. 4 (2003).

65 Sara N. Davison and Gian S. Jhangri, "Existential and religious dimensions of spirituality and their relationship with health-related quality of life in chronic kidney disease," *Clinical Journal of the American Society of Nephrology* 5, no. 11 (2010); Benjamin Ko et al., "Religious beliefs and quality of life in an American inner-city haemodialysis population," *Nephrology Dialysis Transplant* 22, no. 10 (2007); Samir S. Patel et al., "Psychosocial variables, quality of life, and religious beliefs in ESRD patients treated with hemodialysis," *American Journal of Kidney Diseases* 40, no. 5 (2002).

66 Kimmel et al., "ESRD patient quality of life: symptoms, spiritual beliefs, psychosocial factors, and ethnicity": 749.

67 Davison and Jhangri, "Existential and religious dimensions of spirituality and their relationship with health-related quality of life in chronic kidney disease".

5.2.1.1 Perception of satisfaction with life

A link appears to have been established between spirituality and satisfaction with life. [68] Despite the burden of treatment and the constraints imposed by illness, patients will be more inclined to continue with their treatment if their lives still bring them a degree of satisfaction. Al-Arabi identifies three factors that contribute to quality of life: lucidity about the inevitability of loss, strategies to cope with treatments, and a feeling of wellbeing. Spirituality, expressed by the theme of trust in God, is associated with the strategies used to cope with illness. Once again according to Al-Arabi, to assess their quality of life as good, patients must be able to redefine and accept a new identity, as required by the constraints of their illness and treatment.

5.2.1.2 Spirituality and patients' satisfaction with the care received

Spirituality appears to have an influence on the satisfaction felt by patients with regard to the medical care they receive, including their treatment. Hypothetically, this satisfaction should lead to better perseverance with treatment, but despite appearances, this is called into question by several studies.[69] However, it is clear that satisfaction is greater for patients with the greatest religiosity (or extrinsic religion), and this is ascribed by the authors to the fact that the patients appear to be more at ease with rules and authority, a feature of both Churches and healthcare institutions.

5.2.1.3 Spirituality and social support

Some observers believe that it is the social support inherent in the community dimension of religiosity that explains the influence on quality of life.[70] Another study identifies relationships with close family members as the vector for the in-

---

68 Safaa Al-Arabi, "Quality of Life: Subjective," *Nephrology Nursing Journal: Journal of the American Nephrology Nurses' Association* 33, no. 3 (2006); Elisheva Berman et al., "Religiosity in a hemodialysis population and its relationship to satisfaction with medical care, satisfaction with life, and adherence," *American Journal of Kidney Diseases* 44, no. 3 (2004).
69 Berman et al., "Religiosity in a hemodialysis population and its relationship to satisfaction with medical care, satisfaction with life, and adherence"; Mi-K. Song and Laura C. Hanson, "Relationships between psychosocial-spiritual well-being and end-of-life preferences and values in African American dialysis patients," *Journal of Pain and Symptom Management* 38, no. 3 (2009).
70 Patel et al., "Psychosocial variables, quality of life, and religious beliefs in ESRD patients treated with hemodialysis"; Spinale et al., "Spirituality, social support, and survival in hemodialysis patients".

fluence of spirituality on the perception of quality of life.[71] In short, social support makes the link between spirituality and quality of life visible and tangible.

5.2.1.4 Spirituality and psychological wellbeing

The perception of a good quality of life may also be connected to the influence of spirituality on patients' psychological wellbeing. People with a high-quality spiritual life may be less likely to experience episodes of depression or may experience, on average, less intense episodes.[72] According to Davison and Jhangri, "Spirituality promotes psychological adjustment through decreased depression and anxiety, an overall increase in psychological well-being, and greater satisfaction with their role in extended relationships."[73]

5.2.1.5 Spirituality and the feeling of controlling one's life

Last, spirituality may play a role in a sick person's perception of remaining in control of his or her life. Spiritual beliefs may help patients gain and maintain control over their lives when they find a meaningful way to cope with illness and to be happy.[74] In a research project on the self-management of diabetes, the authors showed that spirituality makes a non-negligible contribution, if patients are "believers", to their ability to accept their condition.[75]

5.2.2 Spirituality and pain medicine[76]

All of us experience pain frequently, sometimes on a daily basis, but pain becomes a problem when it is recurrent or even continuous. According to the Amer-

---

71 Al-Arabi, "Quality of Life : Subjective".
72 Berman et al., "Religiosity in a hemodialysis population and its relationship to satisfaction with medical care, satisfaction with life, and adherence"; Sara N. Davison and Gian S. Jhangri, "Existential and supportive care needs among patients with chronic kidney disease," *J Pain Symptom Manage* 40, no. 6 (2010); Patel et al., "Psychosocial variables, quality of life, and religious beliefs in ESRD patients treated with hemodialysis".
73 Sara N. Davison and Gian S. Jhangri, "The relationship between spirituality, psychosocial adjustment to illness, and health-related quality of life in patients with advanced chronic kidney disease," *J Pain Symptom Manage* 45, no. 2 (2013).
74 Al-Arabi, "Quality of Life : Subjective".
75 Rebecca L. Polzer and Margaret S. Miles, "Spirituality in African Americans with diabetes: self-management through a relationship with God," *Qualitative health research* 17, no. 2 (2007).
76 The focus here is on somatic pain and not the existential suffering caused by physical pain.

ican Academy of Pain Medicine, over 100 million Americans experienced chronic pain in 2011.[77] Chronic pain also impacts the economy, since it is estimated to have caused a loss of productivity of between $297 and $335 billion in 2010 in the United States.[78]

As in other sectors of medicine and healthcare, researchers have looked at the role that spirituality and religion could play in the provision of care to manage pain.[79] It goes without saying that this approach to the link between spirituality/religion and pain is not seeking a metaphysical explanation of why pain is present in human lives. Instead, it tries to identify the positive or negative role played by spirituality in the ways in which people cope with chronic or acute pain. The passage below comes from a study by Siddall, Lovell and MacLeod.[80]

The studies reviewed, whether qualitative or quantitative, find no correlation between spiritual life and a mitigation of pain.[81] Instead, the "measurable" effect of the spiritual life of a person suffering from chronic pain lies in the ability to adapt to pain. Here, the influence mechanisms of spirituality identified by the researchers are of various kinds: positive correlations with pain tolerance, with satisfaction with life despite the presence of pain, better strategies for adjusting

---

77 http://www.painmed.org/patientcenter/facts_on_pain.aspx#incidence, retrieved February 2, 2017.

78 http://www.painmed.org/patientcenter/cost-of-pain-to-businesses/#refer, retrieved February 2, 2017.

79 Arndt Büssing et al., "Spiritual needs among patients with chronic pain diseases and cancer living in a secular society," *Pain Medicine* 14, no. 9 (2013); Arndt Büssing et al., "Are spirituality and religiosity resources for patients with chronic pain conditions?," *Pain Medicine* 10, no. 2 (2009); Martin D. Cheatle, "Biopsychosocial Approach to Assessing and Managing Patients with Chronic Pain," *The Medical Clinics of North America* 100, no. 1 (2016); Margaret Feuille and Kenneth I. Pargament, "Pain, mindfulness, and spirituality: A randomized controlled trial comparing effects of mindfulness and relaxation on pain-related outcomes in migraineurs," *Journal of Health Psychology* 20, no. 8 (2015); Alexander Garschagen et al., "Is There a Need for Including Spiritual Care in Interdisciplinary Rehabilitation of Chronic Pain Patients? Investigating an Innovative Strategy," *Pain Practice* 15, no. 7 (2015); Alexander Moreira-Almeida and Harold G. Koenig, "Religiousness and spirituality in fibromyalgia and chronic pain patients," *Current Pain and Headache Reports* 12, no. 5 (2008); Amy B. Wachholtz and Michelle J. Pearce, "Does spirituality as a coping mechanism help or hinder coping with chronic pain?," *Current Pain and Headache Reports* 13, no. 2 (2009); Koenig, Carson, and King, *Handbook of religion and health*, 511–31.

80 Philip J. Siddall, Melanie Lovell, and Rod MacLeod, "Spirituality: What is Its Role in Pain Medicine?," *Pain Medicine* 16, no. 1 (2015).

81 This does not mean that the spiritual experience cannot be a factor in reducing the intensity of pain, but the methodology used in the studies reviewed does not provide much data on the association.

to pain, and better acceptance of pain.[82] The authors conclude with a call for the inclusion of spirituality in the process used to evaluate and treat pain. The benefits reported by the individuals surveyed and the associations identified in the research that support the mobilization of spirituality in pain care are as follows:

> the ability to place and make sense of adversity and to give it a meaningful place within the overall context, direction, or purpose of life can make it easier to endure, particularly if it is seen to be beneficial. Reframing life goals and purpose also allows the formulation of a different direction that still provides a sense of meaningful purpose. Thus, there appears to be growing evidence that addressing issues of spirituality in the person with persistent pain is an important, if not crucial, aspect of managing the pain.[83]

As these illustrations show, the pragmatic approaches are qualified and restricted to the facts that the clinical sciences are able to prove. This type of research is not intended to prove the superiority of a *credo* or demonstrate the existence of God. Pragmatic approaches to spirituality in clinical medicine and the results they produce remain within the limits set by scientificity.

5.3 Conclusion to chapter five

The two pragmatic approaches that preside over the sapientialization of the spiritual experience during illness are similar, although they both have specific features. Whether clinical medicine considers the spiritual experience as a focus of care or as a way to improve the patient's overall state, it does with the goal of providing care, taking the fragility and vulnerability caused by illness into account and, as a result, supporting the joint efforts of caregivers and patients to improve the situation. Whether considered as a "problem" or as a resource, the spiritual experience is integrated into the healthcare project and, as a result, into a logic of treatment (as a focus of care) or instrumentalization (as an adjuvant to care).

In this chapter, as well as the preceding chapter, I have tried to show that the integration of the spiritual experience into a practical approach brings about a substantial change in the reality covered by the term, compared to representations of spirituality in the religious traditions.

---

82 A distinction is made between acceptance of pain and resignation in the presence of pain. In other words, accepting pain does not mean resigning oneself to it.
83 Siddall, Lovell, and MacLeod, "Spirituality: What is Its Role in Pain Medicine?": 7.

The change is wrought by biomedical rationality guided by the task of "vanquishing the 'fatum'",[84] in other words the need to demonstrate and counteract the working of illness, a fatality in the human experience. This form of rationality seeks to master anything that lies outside order, is non-rational or senseless. It also embodies, in its own way, the ethical response to illness, an outpouring of compassion and solidarity for the sick as a way of reassuring them that they still belong to the human and moral community with, and despite, their illness. Because it is part of an order of the world that it discovers and makes manifest, biomedical rationality includes two of the three axes of a wisdom discourse: a search for order in the universe and an ethnical discourse directed towards happiness and a good life.[85]

In fact, the only dimension of a wisdom discourse that is not covered by biomedical rationality is a reflection on the injustices of life and the limits of human reason in order to discover meaning, a discourse known in philosophy and theology as theodicy.[86] This "omission" should not come as a surprise; it reflects the methodological agnosticism that has formed the foundation of medicine since the Hippocratic era and is only strengthened by technoscience, the goals of which are anything but metaphysical. The expression "methodological agnosticism" means that the provision of care is not intended to prove or disprove the existence of an otherworldly being or force that could be called God. From the establishment of Hippocratic medicine in the 4th century B.C., the causes of health and illness were no longer seen as being divine pleasure or anger, but an imbalance in the body's functions.[87] From this standpoint, Hippocratic medicine brought the causes of illness and the restoration of health "back" to Earth, and it could no longer be used to prove the existence of a God or Gods.[88]

The sapientialization of spirituality is therefore the inclusion of the spiritual experience, triggered by illness, in the epistemological and clinical framework of contemporary biomedicine.

84 Dominique Jacquemin, *Bioéthique, médecine et souffrance: jalons pour une théologie de l'échec* (Montréal: Médiaspaul, 2002), 74–75.
85 Crenshaw, "Wisdom Literature". See also chapter 2.
86 The word theodicy is formed from two Greek roots and means, literally, "divine justice" or "the justice of God".
87 See chapter 3.
88 Guy Jobin, *Des religions à la spiritualité. Une appropriation biomédicale du religieux dans l'hôpital*, ed. Eckhard Frick and Cosette Odier, 2nd ed., Soins et spiritualités (Bruxelles: Lumen vitae, 2013[2012]), 84–86.

Because of this, biomedicine alters the characteristic of alterity that marked the spiritual experience in the religious traditions. Alterity is a constitutive element of the spiritual experience in a "religious regime", at least a Christian one, in the sense that spiritual life is given by and comes through an Other. Of course, this is experienced by a person of flesh and blood, who is also unique. Nevertheless it is something that is received, something that is based on a "thing" that is not oneself, something that is based on a part of alterity that is within us and must be welcomed. This alterity retains its otherness in the spiritual experience, since it cannot be controlled or commanded; it makes itself available when it chooses, in the form it chooses: consolation, joy, anger against absurdity, etc. The accounts given by mystics, known and unknown, about this experience show that they have no control over this aspect of their lives. Spiritual life is a donation, whether in the form of a sudden irruption or a quiet growth; it is never a form of mastery.

Biomedicine offers a different anthropological representation, since it sees spiritual life as an object that can be measured, that can be mobilized in adversity, or that can be seen as an internal resource that is intrinsic to human nature.

The next chapter will examine the process of pragmatization that guides the biomedical approach to the spiritual experience, and offer a transition to the second part of the book, which explores another way to address spirituality in the healthcare world.

6 Challenges to sapientialization

The sapientialization of the spiritual experience during illness is a process that is now firmly established, to varying degrees, in healthcare institutions in the Western world. It has led to a *clinical culture* of spirituality that includes a conception of the spiritual experience during illness, an understanding of its role in the care process, and the identification of practices to deal with it. However, despite the undeniable pregnance of the clinical culture in place, it is worth looking at some of the features that remain problematical.

6.1 Some questions

Questions of several different types are raised by the sapientialization of the spiritual experience.

Those concerning professional conduct are the most obvious. The first issue is the involvement of caregivers at each given level of spiritual accompaniment.[1] The clinical culture encourages the care team as a whole to take the patient's spiritual life into account.[2] To what extent should a healthcare professional, other than a chaplain, be involved in the spiritual experience of the patients under his or her care? Is there a limit on the types of interventions the professional should apply? The question is not an idle one—it touches on a vital debate, opposing the promoters of a Hippocratic approach to professional conduct with the supporters of a holistic approach. In short, the debate is between two opposing groups. The first comprises caregivers who consider that, under the ethical principle of doing no harm (*primum, non nocere*), it does not fall within their competence to intervene professionally at the spiritual level. The second includes caregivers who believe that, in keeping with a holistic conception of care, it is their duty to take an interest in the spiritual experience of the patients entrusted to them. The question is one of professional ethics, since the competencies inherently involved

---

1 Cf. section 5.1.2 of chapter 5.
2 Stephen G. Post, Christina M. Puchalski, and David B. Larson, "Physicians and patient spirituality: professional boundaries, competency, and ethics," *Ann Intern Med* 132, no. 7 (2000); Christina M. Puchalski, "Formal and informal spiritual assessment," *Asian Pac J Cancer Prev* 11 Suppl 1 (2010); Christina M. Puchalski, David B. Larson, and Stephen G. Post, "Physicians and Patient Spirituality," *Ann Intern Med* 133, no. 9 (2000); Puchalski et al., "Interdisciplinary spiritual care for seriously ill and dying patients: a collaborative model".

https://doi.org/10.1515/9783110638950-007

in spiritual accompaniment are at the heart of the discussion.[3] A second, equally important, issue faces all members of the care team, and concerns the delicate matter of respect for freedom of religion and freedom of conscience. How far can one go in proposing spiritual activities to patients, now that it has been clearly shown that they have an impact on their physical or mental health?[4] I am referring here to mindfulness, which is recognized in the literature as providing a degree of clinical gain in terms of stress reduction.[5]

Another set of questions concerns the structure of the spiritual accompaniment provided for patients. This is a crucial organizational question. How, within a care institution, will spiritual care be organized? The answer to this question depends on many different factors in each organization and national regime for regulating religious matters in public institutions, in other words the legal space allocated by a state's legislation to religious and spiritual traditions in public life. However, the answer to the question still depends on administrative decisions such as a decision to organize a multi-denominational spiritual accompaniment service, or to rely on the services of volunteers.[6] According to P.-Y.

---

3 Jobin, *Des religions à la spiritualité. Une appropriation biomédicale du religieux dans l'hôpital*, 75–83.
4 Richard P. Sloan, *Blind Faith. The Unholy Alliance of Religion and Medicine* (New York: St. Martin's Press, 2006); Richard P. Sloan and Emilia Bagiella, "Data without a prayer," *Archives of Internal Medicine* 160, no. 12 (2000); Richard P. Sloan and Emilia Bagiella, "Religion and health," *Health Psychology* 20, no. 3 (2001); Richard P. Sloan, Emilia Bagiella, and Thomas Powell, "Religion, spirituality, and medicine," *Lancet* 353, no. 9153 (1999); Richard P. Sloan et al., "Should physicians prescribe religious activities?," *New England Journal of Medicine* 342, no. 25 (2000); Richard P. Sloan and Emilia Bagiella, "Spirituality and medical practice: a look at the evidence," *American Family Physician* 63, no. 1 (2001).
5 Feuille and Pargament, "Pain, mindfulness, and spirituality: A randomized controlled trial comparing effects of mindfulness and relaxation on pain-related outcomes in migraineurs"; Jonathan Greenberg et al., "Mindfulness-based cognitive therapy for depressed individuals improves suppression of irrelevant mental-sets," *Eur Arch Psychiatry Clin Neurosci* 267, no. 3 (2017); Ryan C. Shorey et al., "Dispositional mindfulness, spirituality, and substance use in predicting depressive symptoms in a treatment-seeking sample," *J Clin Psychol* 71, no. 4 (2015).
6 Donia R. Baldacchino, "Nursing competencies for spiritual care," *Journal of Clinical Nursing* 15, no. 7 (2006); Christina M. Puchalski, Stephen G. Post, and Richard P. Sloan, "Physicians and patients' spirituality," *Virtual Mentor* 11, no. 10 (2009); Linda Ross, "Spiritual care in nursing: an overview of the research to date," *Journal of Clinical Nursing* 15, no. 7 (2006); Jackie Smith, "We believe it is better not to explicitly highlight spirituality," *Nursing Standard* 29, no. 37 (2015); Chris Swift, "Omitting spirituality from NMC code disadvantages our patients," *Nursing Standard* 29, no. 38 (2015).

Brandt, there are three recognized ways of organizing spiritual accompaniment:[7] the religious institution model, in which the institution is officially linked to a religious tradition; the model in which an outside religious worker intervenes from time to time at a patient's request or more regularly under contract with the hospital administration; and the model of a chaplaincy integrated into a non-denominational hospital.

The social sciences are also turning their attention to this question.

Sociologically speaking, does the institutionalization of spirituality in care organizations help support the emergence of a new form of mythical or religious thought that structures individuals' relationships with themselves, with others and with the world?[8]

From the point of view of the political sciences, are we seeing the appearance of a new form of the question of meaning, one that matches the secular nature of public institutions in a democracy? Talking about spirituality appears to be tolerated better than talking about religion. The question of meaning, which it does not appear possible to remove from public life, continues to be asked in secularized societies and their secular institutions, but under the guise of spirituality, apparently compatible with the focus on religious neutrality found in many societies. Similarly, but in relation to the structures and power relationships in a healthcare institution, has spirituality, and its control within the institution, become a pawn in the power struggle between the care professions, now that clerical and religious control is on the wane?

Last, from the standpoint of the religious sciences and theology, are we seeing the emergence of a new form of religious discourse for the post-modern world?

There is not room here to answer, exhaustively, all the questions raised by the process involved in the sapientialization of spirituality. Instead, the main focus of this chapter will be to highlight another issue that has not been extensively developed in the contemporary literature. This epistemological problem, inherent to the clinical conceptualization of spirituality, can be expressed succinctly as follows: the clinical sapientialization of spirituality tends to consider spirituality in terms similar to an ethical discourse. My thesis here is that the reception of "spirituality" in the clinical world involves a transfer of language. In-

---

7 Pierre-Yves Brandt, "L'accompagnement spirituel en milieu hospitalier exige-t-il des compétences spécifiques?," in *Spiritualité en milieu hospitalier*, ed. Pierre-Yves Brandt and Jacques Besson (Genève: Labor et Fides, 2015).

8 Liogier, *Souci de soi, conscience du monde: vers une religion globale? [Concern for Oneself, Concern for the World. Toward a Global Religion?]*, 9 – 12.

stead of the traditional religious categories ("salvation", "divinization", "grace", "progression", "mystic", etc.), spirituality is now viewed through another language, the language of virtue ethics, based on accomplishment, self-perfecting, and happiness.[9] Immediately, however, this statement needs to be qualified. What is borrowed from the language of virtue ethics by the biomedical and clinical language of spirituality is its way of understanding the human striving towards ethical perfection and a form of spiritual development. However, it is not the traditional notion of good that drives a person towards spiritual development, but instead the idea of wellbeing, the contemporary visage of happiness and even salvation.

I will examine this thesis in two stages, beginning with a description of wellbeing and self-development. The second stage is a review of the ethics/spirituality distinction in terms of articulation. This approach will introduce the elements needed in the second part of this book, devoted to another way of looking at the spiritual experience during illness.

6.2 Spirituality, wellbeing and ethics[10]

We noted above the pivotal role played by the concept of wellbeing in the clinical language used to describe the spiritual experience during illness.[11] The concept of spirituality is closely connected to the notion of wellbeing, which can be addressed, for research and clinical purposes, by quantitative approaches that measure quality of life.[12]

The association of wellbeing and spirituality is primarily mobilized in a discourse built around the notion of self-accomplishment, meaning that the healthcare world shares a common trait with the world of administration and manage-

---

9 Without being named explicitly, the ethical model of virtue underlying this analysis is the model set out by Aristotle in *Nicomachean Ethics*.

10 This section is taken, with the editor's permission, from an article published in *Interações – Cultura E Comunidade* by PUC Minas, the Pontifical Catholic University of Minas Gerais, Brazil. I thank the journal's editor, Rodrigo Coppe Caldeira for the permission granted: Jobin, "Santé, bien-être et spiritualité: une évaluation critique".

11 Cf. section 5.1.1 of chapter 5.

12 Alain Leplège and Sylvie Duverger, "Qualité de la vie," in *Dictionnaire d'éthique et de philosophie morale*, ed. Monique Canto-Sperber (Paris: Quadrige/Presses universitaires de France, [1996] 2004).

ment,[13] one that crosses institutional boundaries in Western societies and is closely linked with ambient consumerism.

In the healthcare context, self-accomplishment through wellbeing becomes a "task" that can be addressed during illness. This period of time can be seen as a time of "initiative" and "action" by the sick person, setting aside the role of "patient"—someone who endures, who waits, who obeys the orders of illness—to become an "agent", possessing initiative and the ability to do something. Being placed in the position of an agent can be experienced by the patient as a sign of recognition and an opportunity to stand firm and regain a degree of control over the situation. It is, in other words, a form of "empowerment" for a patient for whom everything, in the institutional context, is a reminder of his or her fragility and vulnerability. However, it can also be seen as a discourse that, unknown to the participants, makes sickness or dying a practical time for the production of something as fleeting and immaterial as wellbeing, reconciliation or peace, in short a "productive" time for oneself and for others.

Spiritual self-accomplishment during a time of illness or imminent death is part of what the literature of sociology calls the idea of the good patient or, where applicable, good death, in other words normative conceptions that support the interpretational prejudice of caregivers and which, ultimately, determine the characteristics of the role of "good patient"[14] and the criteria for a "good death". It is clear that this promotion of spiritual self-accomplishment has a connection with the control exercised by biomedicine over the illness experience and the guidelines that determine the conditions and circumstances in which the sick, and their situation, are taken in charge.

After this brief exploration of the question, we can now show the similarity between this discourse and an ethical discourse.

---

13 Pauchant and Forum international sur le management l'éthique et la spiritualité, *Pour un management éthique et spirituel: défis, cas, outils et questions*; Pauchant and Forum international sur le management l'éthique et la spiritualité, *Ethics and spirituality at work: hopes and pitfalls of the search for meaning in organizations*; Mitroff and Denton, *A spiritual audit of corporate America: a hard look at spirituality, religion, and values in the workplace*; Sharda S. Nandram and Margot Esther Borden, *Spirituality and business exploring possibilities for a new management paradigm*, (Berlin: Springer, 2010), http://dx.doi.org/10.1007/978-3-642-02661-4; Freda van der Walt and Jeremias J. de Klerk, "Workplace spirituality and job satisfaction," *Int Rev Psychiatry* 26, no. 3 (2014).
14 Frank, *The Wounded Storyteller. Body, Illness, and Ethics*; Talcott Parsons, *The Social System* (New York: The Free Press, 1951); Kevin White, "Parsons, American Sociology of Medicine and the Sick Role," in *An Introduction to the Sociology of Health and Illness* (Los Angeles, Ca.: Sage, 2009); Graham Scambler, "Deviance, Sick Role and Stigma," in *Sociology as Applied to Medicine*, ed. Graham Scambler (Edimbourg: Saunders Elsevier, 2008).

6.3 Spirituality or ethics? Spirituality or pragmatics?

The scope of the object designated as "spirituality" in present-day biomedical thought, although intended to be comprehensive, is not without ambiguity. One recent criticism is that the definition of spirituality commonly used in palliative care is so similar to the field of humanities in medicine or "the humanist aspect of medicine" that it is fair to ask how the use of the term "spirituality" can designate a specific aspect of the human experience of illness that does not fall into the categories of medical psychology, social psychology, ethics, etc.[15] The answer to this criticism is that although it is true that there may be an overlap between the fields of humanities and spirituality, the term "spirituality" is used to designate the variety of ways in which individuals understand the presence of transcendental meanings in their life.[16] The distinction between spirituality and the humanities, therefore, is based on transcendence. Although this is an important characteristic, it is not entirely satisfactory for my purposes.

6.4 Spirituality and virtue

By refining the above criticism, it is possible to isolate one residual ambiguity, which makes the language of self-accomplishment in contemporary spirituality, and as a result in the biomedical discourse, a calque of ethical discourses such as, for example, virtue ethics.[17] In virtue ethics, an accomplished life is the final cause of actions and work to perfect a moral subject. The accomplishment process is seen as tending towards an ideal of happiness; it results from an effort, a personal striving that mobilizes the energy and will of the moral subject and focuses it on an active and practical search for happiness through acts that make the subject virtuous.

---

15 Pär Salander and Katarina Hamberg, "Why 'Spirituality' Instead of 'The Humanistic Side of Medicine'?," *Academic Medicine* 89, no. 11 (2014).
16 Christina M. Puchalski, Benjamin Blatt, and George Handzo, "In reply to Salander and Hamberg," *Academic Medicine* 89, no. 11 (2014).
17 Bernard Baertschi, "Valeurs et vertus," in *Introduction à l'éthique Penser, croire, agir*, ed. Jean-Daniel Causse and Denis Müller (Genève: Labor et Fides, 2009); Nicolas Dent, "Vertu. Éthique de la vertu," in *Dictionnaire d'éthique et de philosophie morale*, ed. Monique Canto-Sperber (Paris: Quadrige/Presses universitaires de France, 2004); Craig Steven Titus, "Vertus," in *Dictionnaire encyclopédique d'éthique chrétienne*, ed. Laurent Lemoine, Eric Gaziaux, and Denis Müller (Paris: Cerf, 2013).

It is important to emphasize, here, the active and practical aspects of the virtuous search for happiness. It is through the mobilization of the innate dispositions of human beings[18] in actions that virtue achieves its goal and the moral subject gradually approaches the happiness he or she seeks. If a disposition is a "given", in the sense that it is part of human nature, its activation depends on the will of the moral subject and the energy directed towards mobilizing the disposition in concrete actions and a form of life.

There is a clear parallel between the present-day spiritual discourse in the healthcare world and the theory of virtue ethics. The consonance between these two discourses stems from the fact that each deploys a goal of happiness—though defined differently in each case—while also suggesting how this final happiness should be sought, making the quest a task to be accomplished. In addition, the contemporary discourse on spirituality borrows the actual terms used for the psychological manifestation of happiness.

6.5 Both ethical and pragmatic

Another argument can be presented to support the thesis of an ethical understanding of present-day spirituality in the biomedical world. This is a theoretical argument based on the typology of the uses of practical reason proposed by contemporary German philosopher Jürgen Habermas.[19] I want to use this argument to demonstrate the similarity, and in fact the strong resemblance, between the spiritual discourse in the clinical world and current ethical categories. However, we must start with an incursion into the theory.

Practical reason is the part of rational human capacity involved in all transactions with the word in the mode of action. Practical rationality is at the heart of all deliberation and action. This ancient notion, repeated in medieval philosophy and theology, has been "revisited" by Habermas who identifies three ways in which practical reason is exercised: "Different tasks are required of practical reason under the aspects of the purposive, the good, and the just. Correspondingly, the constellation of reason and volition changes [...]"[20] The uses are, respectively, the pragmatic (purposive), the ethical (good), and the moral (just) uses of practical reason. Here, I will discuss only the first two uses, which see

---

18 For Aristotle, virtue stems from a disposition. Aristote, *Éthique de Nicomaque*, trans. Jean Voilquin (Paris: Gallimard Flammarion, 1992), 60.
19 Jürgen Habermas, "De l'usage pragmatique, éthique et moral de la raison pratique," in *De l'éthique de la discussion*, ed. Jürgen Habermas, Champs (Paris: Flammarion, 1992).
20 Habermas, "De l'usage pragmatique, éthique et moral de la raison pratique": 96.

action from the standpoint of an active subject, while the third use (the just) necessarily involves the moral or third-person point of view, in other words a perspective that goes beyond personal motivations for action, however sublime.

The defining characteristic of the pragmatic use of practical reason is the choice of means applied to a given goal. This is "purposive rationality, its goal being to discover appropriate techniques, strategies, or programs."[21] We are in the realm of instrumental rationality, in its relationship with the physical world, and strategic rationality, when a pragmatic use is applied to relationships with others. In both cases, the other (object or person) is considered as a means to be used or manipulated to achieve the goals set by the agent.

Ethical use of practical reason concerns existential decisions about a good life, which involve a relationship between the subject and a set of values that the subject considers to be fundamental. These values provide a measure of the good life targeted, which structures the life that the moral subject would like to lead. We are at the innermost part of an understanding of oneself and one's personal identity. The quest for happiness is a form of self-accomplishment and self-development that, according to Habermas, comes under the ethical use of practical reason since existential choices are motivated by a desire to incarnate the ideal presiding over one's personal life project and since the criteria for discerning the direction and rightness of the actions chosen also relate to an ideal. As emphasized by Habermas after Charles Taylor, the ethical mode of practical reason relates to "strong evaluations,"[22] the criteria used to make a moral judgment in terms of good/bad, better/worse and higher/lower, which "take their orientation from a goal posited absolutely for me, that is, from the highest good of a self-sufficient form of life that has its value in itself."[23]

6.6 Criticism of the identification of spirituality with ethics

In short, whether we use the "old" theory of virtue ethics or mobilize Habermas's theory of practical rationality, it is clear, to me, that the contemporary humanist spiritual discourse reuses (possibly unconsciously) the categories of an ethical discourse, which raises questions for anyone who knows even a little about the religious spiritual traditions.

---

21 Habermas, "De l'usage pragmatique, éthique et moral de la raison pratique": 97.
22 Charles Taylor, *Sources of the Self. The Making of the Modern Identity* (Cambridge, Ma: Harvard University Press, 1989), 4.
23 Habermas, "De l'usage pragmatique, éthique et moral de la raison pratique": 99.

I have already mentioned the reframing of the spiritual discourse using the parameters of virtue ethics, such as self-development. What I would like to emphasize now is the issue of spiritual experience as a production, and even an emanation, of the subject. After a brief description of this voluntarist conception, I will compare it to another conception of spiritual life.

The contemporary spiritual discourse, taken up by a large number of biomedical theoreticians, strongly emphasizes the subject's effort and work in the spiritual dynamic. The individual and his or her resources are at the heart of spiritual life and, in the event of spiritual distress, at the heart of the recovery process. Calls for the mobilization of spirituality in terms of "resources", "energy" and "locus of control"[24] are frequently found in the biomedical literature. As a result, spiritual resources are considered and thought of as the basic material of the spiritual experience, available to the subject and necessary for the path towards self-development and wellbeing. The resources are considered to form part of every human being and of his or her intrinsic nature.

On the other hand, the Christian religious traditions make grace the "motor" of spiritual life. Grace is a gift; it cannot be deserved, since it is a pure gratuity from the Other. One possible objection to this conception of grace as a gratuitous gift is that the religious spiritual traditions have set up a panoply of practical ways to make it possible to receive the gift, including ascetic practices that require the subject's voluntary adhesion. Here, as in virtue ethics, an effort is required on the part of the subject, an implementation and mobilization of will

---

24 Andrea D. Clements et al., "RSAS-3: validation of a very brief measure of Religious Commitment for use in health research," *J Relig Health* 54, no. 1 (2015); Katrina J. Debnam et al., "Spiritual health locus of control and health behaviors in African Americans," *Am J Health Behav* 36, no. 3 (2012); Sadaaki Fukui, Vincent R. Starnino, and Holly B. Nelson-Becker, "Spiritual wellbeing of people with psychiatric disabilities: the role of religious attendance, social network size and sense of control," *Community Ment Health J* 48, no. 2 (2012); Godfrey Gregg, "I'm a Jesus girl: coping stories of Black American women diagnosed with breast cancer," *J Relig Health* 50, no. 4 (2011); Anne-C. Hornborg, "Designing rites to re-enchant secularized society: new varieties of spiritualized therapy in contemporary Sweden," *J Relig Health* 51, no. 2 (2012); Michael J. Lowis, Anthony C. Edwards, and Mary Burton, "Coping with retirement: well-being, health, and religion," *J Psychol* 143, no. 4 (2009); Michael E. McCullough and Brian L. Willoughby, "Religion, self-regulation, and self-control: Associations, explanations, and implications," *Psychol Bull* 135, no. 1 (2009); Larry W. Redmond, "Spiritual coping tools of religious victims of childhood sexual abuse," *J Pastoral Care Counsel* 68, no. 1–2 (2014); Collin A. Ross, "Talking about God with Trauma Survivors," *Am J Psychother* 70, no. 4 (2016); Donna E. Stewart and Tracy Yuen, "A systematic review of resilience in the physically ill," *Psychosomatics* 52, no. 3 (2011); Benita Walton-Moss, Ellen M. Ray, and Kathleen Woodruff, "Relationship of spirituality or religion to recovery from substance abuse: a systematic review," *J Addict Nurs* 24, no. 4 (2013).

in the ascetic exercise. However, asceticism, understood in this way, *does not produce grace*. Ascetic practices are understood in theology as being preparation of the "ground" to receive grace from the Other. Work and effort play an important role in the spiritual experience lived and interpreted in terms of the gift, but are not its prime cause or effective cause.

In addition to the reframing of spirituality in the categories of self-development and ethics, we must consider a voluntarist conception of the spiritual experience. But placing spiritual experience under the aegis of a voluntarist strategy to produce meaning is also related to pragmatic rationality, like the mobilization of spiritual resources in a physical or mental recovery process. This is reflected in the biomedical and clinical literature on the topic. A number of studies have emphasized the therapeutic profit that can be derived from considering the spiritual experience of patients. One example of this type of research is seen in the field of pain medicine, where a recent survey of the literature shows the positive and significant correlation between the intensity of a patient's spiritual life and his or her perception of quality of life, despite the continual presence of pain.[25]

The fact remains that the strategy selected by the biomedical literature, to reframe the spiritual experience in the mode of means-ends rationality,[26] derives from a particular way of considering human beings. This is the anthropology of *homo faber*, the productive human being. And without any pejorative connotation, this view of human spiritual dynamics could be called Promethean. However, this is not the only way to address the question. Spirituality and ethics can be linked, while maintaining their separate integrity and preserving the interpretation of spiritual experience as a participation in the dynamic of a gift, without burying it in the dynamic of production. This other option is to consider an *articulation* between spirituality and ethics, rather than an *alignment of spirituality on ethics*.

6.7 A proposal for articulation

The articulation of ethics and spirituality is not gratuitous or opportunistic—for example, because spirituality happens to be in fashion—or a denominational attempt to regain control on the discussion about spirituality. As I have suggested,

---

25 Siddall, Lovell, and MacLeod, "Spirituality: What is Its Role in Pain Medicine?". Cf. section 5.2.2 of chapter 5.
26 Guy Jobin, "La spiritualité: facteur de résistance au pouvoir biomédical de soigner ?," *Revue d'éthique et de théologie morale* 266, no. HS (2011): 140.

the recent history of Western healthcare institutions and a theoretical reflection based on clinical experience both support articulation.

6.7.1 Recent history[27]

Ethics and spirituality are brought into contact in the healthcare world for historical reasons. The institutionalization of bioethics in the clinical and research sectors in the Western world laid the groundwork for the institutionalization of biomedical interest in the spiritual experience of patients, as shown by several different examples.

First, it is important to remember that the secular bioethics movement that emerged in the 1960s and 1970s was initially carried forward by various theologians or philosophers who did not hide their interest in religious matters. The names of Paul Ramsey, Bernard Häring, James Childress, Edmund Pellegrino and André Hellegers are all associated with the early stages of bioethics in the United States.[28]

Second, the institutionalization of bioethics occurred in an interdisciplinary setting, in which theology was able to carve out its own place while respecting the secularity of the project as a whole.[29] The theological discourse was able to

---

27 This section repeats elements from Jobin, "Development of the Connection Between Spirituality and Medicine: Historical and Current Issues in Clinics".

28 Tom L. Beauchamp and James F. Childress, *Principles of Biomedical Ethics*, 7th ed. (Oxford: Oxford University Press, 2012); Bernard Häring, *Medical Ethics* (Notre Dame, Ind.: Fides, 1973); Edmund D. Pellegrino, John Langan, and John Collins Harvey, *Catholic perspectives on medical morals: foundational issues* (Dordrecht: Kluwer Academic Publishers, 1989); Paul Ramsey, *The Patient as Person* (New Haven: Yale University Press, 1970); Edmund D. Pellegrino and David C. Thomasma, *For the patient's good: the restoration of beneficence in health care* (New York: Oxford University Press, 1988).

29 Lisa S. Cahill, "Bioethics, theology, and social change," *J Relig Ethics* 31, no. 3 (2003); Alastair V. Campbell, "Secularised bioethics and the passion of religion," *New Rev Bioeth* 1, no. 1 (2003); Roberto Dell'Oro, "Theological discourse and the postmodern condition: the case of bioethics," *Med Health Care Philos* 5, no. 2 (2002); Marcio F. Dos Anjos and Hubert F. Lepargneur, "Bioethics and Christian theology in Brazil," *J Int Bioéthique* 19, no. 1–2 (2008); Scott J. Fitzpatrick et al., "Religious Perspectives on Human Suffering: Implications for Medicine and Bioethics," *J Relig Health* 55, no. 1 (2016); Kevin W. Wildes, "Religion in bioethics: a rebirth," *Christ Bioeth* 8, no. 2 (2002); Laurie Zoloth, "Religion and the public discourse of bioethics," *Med Ethics* (Burlingt Mass) (1999); Brenda Margaret Appleby and Nuala P. Kenny, "Relational personhood, social justice and the common good: Catholic contributions toward a public health ethics," *Christian Bioethics* 16, no. 3 (2010); Andrea Vicini, "La loi morale naturelle: perspectives internationales pour la réflexion bioéthique contemporaine," *Transversalités* 122 (2012); Andrea Vici-

make a critical, but not apologetic, contribution to secular bioethics. For example, theologians showed that theological questioning could break down religiously-inspired medical approaches to morality—founded on permission and prohibition—by making the meaning of actions or a focus on human vulnerability and fragility major elements in the bioethical reflection.[30]

Third, several authorities responsible for the bioethical regulation of clinical actions, research, and public health policy, were open to contributions from people associated with religious and spiritual traditions. For example, in France, the national advisory committee on ethics for life sciences and health (Comité consultatif national d'éthique pour les sciences de la vie et de la santé, or CCNE) included among its members representatives from various philosophic and spiritual families. In North America, chaplains sat on a number of hospital ethics committees.

Fourth, bioethics and spirituality had some thematic similarities, including the crucial issue of the humanization of healthcare institutions. Whether to humanize care relationships, often reduced to technical gestures or dry expertise, or the management and culture of highly bureaucratic organizations, ethics and spirituality were often called on to found criticism (sometimes severe, but always constructive) of the underlying trend towards dehumanization in the Western care traditions.

Fifth, and last, in the clinical practice of spiritual accompaniment, it was not unusual for ethical issues to be raised in connection with the moral standards in effect in a specific religious tradition. In the other direction, religious questions could be found at the core of the clinical approach of ethical discernment.

In short, in the clinical field, ethics and religion/spirituality have been close neighbours since the mid-20th century. The institutionalization of these two approaches to illness, and the consequences of institutionalization, have made it possible to build the bridges mentioned above. These are situational bridges that, to use the words of sociologist Renée C. Fox speaking about bioethics, result from a double "happening": the events occurred more or less spontaneously, with no specific plan, and were structured by circumstances and locations and in response to new, unprecedented "needs".

---

ni, "Respecting life: theology and bioethics," *Journal of the Society of Christian Ethics* 35, no. 1 (2015).

30 There are, of course, various religious discourses that draw on bioethics. The literature includes proposals for Christian bioethics, Jewish bioethics, etc. It would be better, in these cases, to speak of the morality of religious care, since bioethics is primarily a secular endeavour. As a result, there is a contradiction in the terms, and in the reflective exercise, with the expression "denominational bioethics".

However, the articulation between spirituality and ethics is not justified solely by institutional arrangements. By offering a theoretical exploration of the nature of care, it shows that the link between the two is founded on the logic inherent in the support provided for the sick. This task of examining the articulation between ethics and spirituality has been taken on by Belgian ethicist and theologian Dominique Jacquemin.

6.7.2 The articulation inherent in the nature of the care provided for the sick

Dominique Jacquemin's examination of the complex links between ethics and spirituality begins with the phenomenon of suffering and the questions it raises for all the individuals involved in the care relationship.[31] The real, difficult and always destabilizing experience of suffering is opposed here to the theoretical discourse on self-accomplishment. Far from being a dolorist apology, Jacquemin's thesis considers suffering as a "place to think, […] and to apprehend what it tells us about that which is human."[32]

One of the goals of medicine is to relieve the pain and suffering caused by illness.[33] However, suffering is a paradox in the sense that it is simultaneously an existential enigma—what is the point of suffering?[34]—and a place for "revealing the humanity"[35] of the person who suffers. We can go even further and describe suffering as the "moment of anthropological revelation" when the complexity of the human being and of the interconnections between its constituent dimensions are unveiled.

---

31 Dominique Jacquemin, *Quand l'autre souffre. Éthique et spiritualité*, Donner raison (Bruxelles: Lessius, 2010). The work of François Yumba on the concept of spirituality in the work of Dominique Jacquemin should also be noted. François Yumba, *Les patients perdus de vue dans la prise en charge du Sida. Articulation entre santé, spiritualité et salut à partir de leur vécu à Kinshasa*, ed. Gilles Routhier, Théologies pratiques (Bruxelles: Lumen vitae, 2017), 47–50. My understanding differs from the analysis of F. Yumba, since I focus on the articulation between ethics and spirituality in Jacquemin's work.
32 Jacquemin, *Quand l'autre souffre. Éthique et spiritualité*, 10.
33 "The Goals of Medicine: Setting New Priorities. Special Supplement".
34 This is a question that goes beyond a functional explanation of pain as a physiological alert mechanism, defined as an "An unpleasant sensory and emotional experience associated with actual or potential tissue damage, or described in terms of such damage", cf. Association for the Study of Pain International, "IASP Taxonomy." International Association for the Study of Pain, http://www.iasp-pain.org/Education/Content.aspx?ItemNumber=1698&navItemNumber=576.
35 Jacquemin, *Quand l'autre souffre. Éthique et spiritualité*, 10.

In Jacquemin's view, the support provided by clinicians to accompany suffering can be deployed along two separate but complementary axes: ethics and spirituality.

Ethics is defined as "a practice that accompanies medical decisions in a hospital environment and a key way to set up a space to compare the various points of view that coexist within the hospital about the ethical questions raised."[36] Ethics must meet the requirements of a process guided by reason, the fundamental pillar for discerning how to do the right thing at a time of uncertainty and questioning. Ethics in the healthcare world is a reflective timeout, in other words a place and a time where it is possible to step back from the immediateness of practices and decisions. Using prudential judgment, the reflective timeout has several stages:

> the goal is to find out more about the situation, to assess it lucidly both in terms of its actual content and the issues it involves; to remember that the analysis of a situation from an ethical point of view is not possible without invoking an external element in the form of the "standards" of a moral or religious code, in other words a tradition; and last, to apply a dynamic approach where a "straight aim" is important while remaining dependant on a sometimes paradoxical relationship between the abruptness of the situation and the ideal aim of the principles.[37]

However, we must go beyond this definition to look at the actual conditions for the institutionalization of ethical concerns in healthcare establishments, which has guided reflections in the clinical world by limiting them, according to Jacquemin, "to the critical, rational, decision- and action-related dimension alone."[38] And, we could add, when they are not reduced to a conduct-related review—quasi-judicial in nature—on what is permitted or forbidden. Suffering, because of what it imposes on patients and triggers among caregivers, leads to broader questions than the rationality of a given action. Those questions are: "Who am I? What am I experiencing? What is the meaning of illness?"[39]

This is why ethics is necessary, but not sufficient to deal with the existential questions that accompany serious illness, chronic illness and dying. Ethics is not

---

36 Jacquemin, *Quand l'autre souffre. Éthique et spiritualité*, 104. The author borrows this definition from his colleague Pierre Boitte.
37 Dominique Jacquemin, *La bioéthique et la question de Dieu: une voie séculière d'intériorité et de spiritualité?* (Montréal: Médiaspaul, 1996), 44.
38 Jacquemin, *Quand l'autre souffre. Éthique et spiritualité*, 10 – 11.
39 Jacquemin, *Quand l'autre souffre. Éthique et spiritualité*, 58; 156.

enough to accompany a suffering person, even if illness provides a time of choice[40] deliberation and discernment.

By providing a broad definition of spirituality, Jacquemin aims to go beyond a merely ethical perspective. Spirituality is "a movement involving the bodily, psychological, ethical and religious dimensions; the movement of the dimensions and their recognition by the subject defining 'the spiritual dimension'."[41] He adds that

> the spiritual dimension is related to that which shapes the dynamic of an existence, a dynamic that is present in each person and places him or her against a horizon that gives a plenitude of meaning to his or her life experiences. [...] The spiritual dimension of human life must be considered in terms of the quality and unity of the being, the totality of the movement that bears its existence, while the movement itself is borne by the pace of the illness.[42]

In this way, the spiritual dimension acts as a force that resists the fragmentation of the subject brought about by both the illness itself and, it must be admitted, the technoscience used in providing care. Spirituality can play this role of reunification because, in Jacquemin's view, it is broader that the ethical and religious dimensions. It encompasses them, not as a higher-level dimension, but as the guiding force for the integration of the dimensions into human life. And this is the level affected by the destabilizing forces of suffering.

In short, Jacquemin's proposal is based on a precise anthropological representation used to support the thesis that spiritual issues go beyond the necessary, but narrow ethical perspective. The focus on spirituality makes it possible to delve more deeply into the condition of a suffering human being. As a result, spirituality is not something that is superimposed on the care relationship—instead, it is an essential "cog" in the process. It is what a frank examination of suffering reveals. Spirituality is not a "plus" or an "elsewhere" of care practices. On the contrary, the ethical and spiritual perspectives are "connatural":

> Can ethical reflection not be legitimately understood as a place, an approach, and a space for the spiritual dimension, which lies at the heart of every existence? [...] In terms of a possible link between ethics and spirituality, we see it, without veering into apologetics, as a service that ethics could render to both society and spirituality: to not make spirituality a "non-place" for practices or a space that is inaccessible to rational exercise, to the point

---

40 Jacquemin, *Quand l'autre souffre. Éthique et spiritualité*, 10.
41 Jacquemin, *Quand l'autre souffre. Éthique et spiritualité*, 12–13.
42 Jacquemin, *Quand l'autre souffre. Éthique et spiritualité*, 59.

that any possibility for affirmation or recognition within our social, persona or professional universe, both individual and collective, is excluded.[43]

More specifically, Jacquemin discusses the articulation between ethics and spirituality by explaining its three basic operations: openness to questioning about meaning, support for the question of suffering, and a focus on actions.[44] First, discussions that must be successfully completed, decisions that must be made, actions that must be taken, and consequences that must be assumed: these unavoidable elements in an ethical examination touch on the foundations of what constitutes the meaning of a life, for both the sick person and the caregiver. Ethical questions lead to questions about meaning. Next, the care relationship, a relationship of support, becomes even more significant when it takes place in a climate of mutual recognition between the patient, in the intimacy of his or her suffering, and the caregiver, able to identify the repercussions of the other person's suffering on his or her own professional life. Last, the ethics/spirituality articulation makes it possible to launch a critical review of the conditions in which care is provided. Although it is a concrete, active response to a request for relief, care is also a element in the response made by a human being (and humanity itself) to vital, and never fully resolved, questions about the meaning of suffering, sickness and death.

In short, "the ethical path as a critical, rational space for argument may contribute not only to the recognition of contemporary spirituality, but also to its being taken into account as a constitutive dimension of the caregiving responsibility."[45]

6.8 Conclusion to chapter six

Dominique Jacquemin's proposal distinguishes between ethics and spirituality. It is based on three pillars: 1) ethics as an access route to spiritual questioning; 2) spirituality as a way to reveal the limits of ethical questioning strictly centred on a narrow conception of rationality; and 3) the connaturality of ethics and spirituality from an anthropological point of view, as shown by the experience of suffering. This thesis is clearly different from the consensual discourse supporting the equivalence of spirituality and ethics. However, it also mobilizes the

---

43 Jacquemin, *Quand l'autre souffre. Éthique et spiritualité*, 146.
44 Jacquemin, *Quand l'autre souffre. Éthique et spiritualité*, 148–52.
45 Jacquemin, *Quand l'autre souffre. Éthique et spiritualité*, 160.

framework for the sapientialization of spirituality, as described in Part One. In fact, Jacquemin considers the articulation from the standpoint of contemporary medicine.[46]

The fact that spiritual questioning during illness could add an extra load to the technoscientific approach to sickness (a constituent part of which appears to be concrete ethical support) is seen as something that could challenge the care dynamic from the inside. Jacquemin is rightly critical of the danger of spirituality being instrumentalized by the biomedical approach.[47] But the conception of spirituality that underlies his examination remains influenced by the sapiential posture that prevails in the biomedical world, the bioethical world and among many analysts in the field of "spirituality and health". We must, at the same time, recognize that Jacquemin's critical work is part of a thought process that is legitimate within both the healthcare world—founding criticism of the effects of technoscientific care on a fundamental theory and experience of care that draws support from normative anthropology—and in the world of theological reflection on care practices. This work makes it possible to address the actual problems that arrive in the clinical sector using the framework of a philosophy of care.

None of this prevents us from using another, equally legitimate analytical and critical posture to reflect on the issues raised by the spiritual experience during illness. This posture takes a fresh look at the situation by taking into account and criticizing the dynamics and normative logic that run through the healthcare world and determine the approach to the spiritual experience. Here, our attention will be focused on the spiritual experience rather than on a theory of care. This approach will highlight other issues with greater potential for conflict than those that appear in the sapiential approach.

---

46 "We intend to show [...] that we must think today about a link between ethics and spirituality in order to assess, at the heart of contemporary medicine, as extensively as possible, the relationship between professionals and patients and the reality of suffering, so that suffering can be recognized and supported as required, in other words without a diminution or excess of responsibility." Dominique Jacquemin, "La confrontation avec la souffrance: un lieu pour penser le lien entre éthique et spiritualité," in *Spiritualité: interpellation et enjeux pour le soin et la médecine*, ed. Danièle Leboul and Dominique Jacquemin, Les carnets de l'espace éthique de Bretagne occidentale (Montpellier: Sauramps médical, 2010): 53.
47 Jacquemin, *Quand l'autre souffre. Éthique et spiritualité*, 60; 157.

Part II. **The "subversive" nature of spirituality in healthcare**

7 Questions relating to spiritual anthropology

As mentioned at the end of the preceding chapter, the approach in the remaining portion of the book will be to reflect on spiritual experience during illness in a way that differs from the biomedical and clinical method described in Part One. For this purpose I will use the path set out by spiritual anthropology, a discourse that results from the effort made by human beings to understand themselves from a spiritual point of view. Spiritual anthropology is a theory about human beings' spiritual "nature", the inherent characteristics of this aspect of human life and its "functions", operations, repercussions on individual and collective life, etc. Discussing spiritual anthropology involves tracing the spiritual experience back to its most fundamental and least exposed "places." I believe this is necessary because the biomedical and clinical approach to the spiritual experience is based on a form of spiritual anthropology that appears paradoxical: its discourse diminishes the important of crucial elements of the spiritual experience which nevertheless structure it and give it life, like any other discourse on the spiritual experience. These elements, which are part of every spiritual experience but rarely addressed in themselves and in the role they play are: language, tradition and group. Their importance will be discussed in the first section of this chapter.

The second section looks at another aspect of the spiritual anthropology of the biomedical discourse, which I have called the "materiality" of spiritual life. This quality of spiritual life is brought into play by the discussion of the source and "location" of the spiritual experience of human beings. Where does the spiritual experience come from? What is its source? These questions are not just theoretical; they influence the way in which we try to understand the interactions between the spiritual life, psychological life and corporeal life of human beings.

It is important to specify why I identify language, tradition, the group and the "materiality" of spiritual life as matters for discussion and for a critique of the spiritual anthropology underling the biomedical and clinical discourse. The relevance of these analysis categories becomes more evident when we consider how the biomedical spiritual discourse is constructed. Like other contemporary spiritual discourses, it is partly built using a process of *de-traditionalization*, a term that designates the process of extracting one or more elements from an oral, written, practical or other tradition. Like a loan, the element is taken out of the network of meaning for which it was a hub in the original tradition. In the world of healthcare and therapy, the de-traditionalization process can take one of two forms.

https://doi.org/10.1515/9783110638950-008

First, the process is operationalized when elements from pre-existing religious or spiritual traditions are extracted from their original symbolic system and ordered for a different purpose. One obvious example is yoga, a Hindu tradition with an ascetic function,[1] that in the Western world has acquired a "therapeutic" function for stress relief.[2] Another example is mindfulness, from the Vietnamese Buddhist tradition, which has also become a stress reduction strategy.[3]

Second, de-traditionalization is part of the search for a universal definition of spirituality. The goal is to identify a common spiritual denominator for all the religious and spiritual traditions. This common denominator, postulated as being present in all traditions and crossing all ideological and denominational boundaries, will be identified as "spirituality."[4]

De-traditionalization therefore raises the question of the relationship that a spiritual discourse maintains with the world (through language), with a tradition of thought, and with a reference group. The de-traditionalization process masks the fact that every spiritual phenomenon lies in the realm of language, is still part of a tradition—whichever one it is—and has a social dimension. Far from being anodyne details, the concepts of language, tradition and group highlight the anthropological presuppositions that give life to de-traditionalization as mobilized to build the biomedical and clinical discourse on spirituality.

7.1 Language

At first sight, language, whether spoken or written, has all the characteristics of an instrument, appearing to be a tool that supports the transmission of thought. In this instrumental representation, thought, emotions, and affect, in short, all the impulses that occur in the innermost being, precede speech and writing,

---

1 Gerald James Larson and Ram S. Bhattacharya, *Yoga: India's philosophy of meditation*, 1st ed. (Delhi: Motilal Banarsidass Publishers, 2008). In general, ascetics refers to a set of practices that target detachment from worldly realities. In several religious or spiritual traditions, ascetics is part of each individual's maturation.
2 Arndt Büssing et al., "Yoga as a therapeutic intervention," *Evid Based Complement Alternat Med* 2012 (2012); Laura Douglass, "Thinking through the body: the conceptualization of yoga as therapy for individuals with eating disorders," *Eat Disord* 19, no. 1 (2011); Lila Louie, "The effectiveness of yoga for depression: a critical literature review," *Issues Ment Health Nurs* 35, no. 4 (2014); Shivarama Varambally and Bengaluru N. Gangadhar, "Yoga: a spiritual practice with therapeutic value in psychiatry," *Asian J Psychiatr* 5, no. 2 (2012).
3 *Kabat-Zinn, Au coeur de la tourmente, la pleine conscience.*
4 We saw, in chapter 4, that universality is seen as a characteristic of spirituality.

which are physical traces that can be heard or read. Language is considered to be a soundboard for the expression of the inner impulses of human beings, or else a transmission belt. However, this conception of language is reductionist, because it reduces the human gift of language to the rank of a communication skill. The attention focused on communication (meaning the dissemination or transfer of information) may hide the fact that language is fundamental and is in fact the matrix for our relationship to the world. In more direct terms, language influences the manner in which people see and understand the world around them, which is more fundamental than simply conveying information. Therefore from a conceptual point of view, we must distinguish between language, as a medium for our relationship to the world, and speech (or language) as a medium of communication.[5]

The influence of language on our perception of the world is shown in the following example, where the same reality has two utterly different aspects, depending on whether it is perceived through the language of science or the language of everyday life. The two languages are illustrated here by Austrian writer Robert Musil:

> A barometric low hung over the Atlantic. It moved eastward toward a high-pressure area over Russia without as yet showing any inclination to bypass this high in a northerly direction. The isotherms[6] and isotheres[7] were functioning as they should. The air temperature was appropriate to the annual mean temperature and to the aperiodic monthly fluctuations of the temperature. [...] The water vapour in the air was at its maximal state of tension, while the humidity was minimal. In a word that characterises the facts fairly accurately, even if it is a bit old-fashioned: it was a fine day in August 1913.[8]

The contrast between the scientific-objective description (barometric low, isotherm, isothere, annual mean temperature, aperiodic monthly fluctuation, etc.) and the subjective words "fine day" provide an eloquent example, showing how language directs not only our choice of words, but more profoundly the very way in which we view an occurrence. The factual scientific description is not intended to provide an assessment or a value judgment about the relationship between the air temperature and the annual mean, while the "fine day"

---

5 This is why language is not confined to words, but includes non-verbal signs such as gestures. I use the term "language" here in its broad sense.

6 Imaginary line joining points at the same temperature.

7 Imaginary line joining points at the same mean summer temperature.

8 Robert Musil, *L'homme sans qualités*, tome 1 (traduction Philippe Jacottet), Paris, Seuil, 1966, p. 9, cited *in* Jean Greisch, *L'âge herméneutique de la raison* (Paris: Éditions du Cerf, 1985), 33. English excerpt from Robert Musil, *The Man Without Qualities*, translated by Sophie Wilkins.

comment is a value judgment. The language choice has epistemological value, because it influences the way of knowing. It is clear that language is not limited to a choice of appropriate words, in this case belonging to science and meteorology, but also involves tools and methodologies also belonging to science that underlie an objective knowledge of the occurrence. In addition, only "everyday" language can be used to state that the day was "fine", based on the criteria of the person concerned, drawn from his or her life experience.

This trivial example shows that language orients our relationship to the world. A scientific relationship to the world generates perception and knowledge that differ from those generated by an everyday relationship. In other words, language mediates our relationship to the world.

Let us return to our topic. Language—in the fundamental sense used here—unavoidably mediates the spiritual experience. Without language there is no access to the spiritual experience. This statement loses its banality when it is applied to both the language that mediates the spiritual experience of the person describing it and to the language the orients knowledge of the spiritual experience of others. Caregivers and chaplains can only have access to the spiritual experience of a patient through the language he or she uses to describe it. Similarly, the clinical language used to describe the spiritual experience is the filter through which the caregiver "reads" the spiritual experience described.[9] In short, there can only ever be mediated access to the spiritual experience of another person.

To examine this question in more depth, I will use the work of Michel de Certeau to argue in favour of a spiritual anthropology that addresses the fundamental issue of language.[10]

In the second volume of *La fable mystique*, published in 2013 in an edition edited by Luce Giard, de Certeau devotes a chapter to the "Uses of tradition." Discussing a search for a founding spiritual experience in the writing of a spiritual author, in this case John of the Cross, de Certeau states:

> All spiritual experience that expresses itself, the moment it is expressed, is "alienated", so to speak, in language. First, it uses the words of others; it therefore is subject to the concomitant constraints. John of the Cross, Surin, or the man of today speaks only a language received from others. The words—and their laws—cannot be freely invented. They are

9 I have already pointed out that present-day clinical language "divides" the spiritual reality into categories that hide several segments of the spiritual experience during illness. Readers are referred to the discussion of the terms "need" and "desire" (chapter 5, section 5.1.1.2.)
10 The rest of this chapter is based on the argument set out in my article Guy Jobin, "Quelle anthropologie pour inclure la dimension spirituelle aux soins? Perspectives d'avenir," *Revue théologique de Louvain* 48, no. 4 (2017): 510–34.

"given" to experience, which does not exist anywhere else than where it is said. Moreover, that expression is submitted to an "obligatory passage", namely, the triage and pressure of a group. Its only existence is by leave of the passport issued by the community in which it is accepted. Spiritual literature shows this in a thousand and one ways. Strictly speaking there is no such thing as an individual experience. That is a mirage. [...] A spiritual writing gives only the "I" of experience taken in the "we" of a language; from this point of view, the author or the subject appears only as already subjected to the law of a community. This is what makes his experience into a language. Every writing is therefore of an "ecclesial" structure.[11]

It goes without saying that de Certeau's comments primarily concern spiritual texts, but also apply to oral messages and spiritual discourses.[12] It is also important to note that the last word in this extract must be understood in a broad sense. The word "ecclesial" highlights the fact that spiritual writing belongs inevitably to a community of discourses that provides an interpretative framework[13] for anyone who says anything about his or her spiritual experience.

This is a strong position that contradicts generally accepted ideas about spiritual life, at least those that are part of our common culture. De Certeau insists on the language-based nature of the spiritual experience and on the influence of the community (or group) on the experience itself. I will return to this second aspect below.

It is clear to de Certeau that language is not a *neutral* means of communication of intimate, and in this spiritual, experiences; it is first and foremost a medium for recording the experience in the thickness and texture of reality. The "experience [...] does not exist anywhere else than where it is said."[14] Experience exists in the space opened up by language. This leads to the conclusion that language is not simply a sounding board for our innermost experiences, but should be seen as a locus where experience becomes embodied—through speech or writing—and as a locus that structures the actual experience.

Language is therefore the passport of experience. Its function as a "vector" is clearly identifiable in the care environment. In addition to the points mentioned

11 Michel de Certeau, *La fable mystique II. XVIe-XVIIe siècle*, Bibliothèque des histoires (Paris: Gallimard, 2013), 166–67.
12 Dominique Salin, *L'expérience spirituelle et son langage: leçons sur la tradition mystique chrétienne* (Paris: Éditions des facultés jésuites de Paris, 2015), 95–119.
13 These are prejudices of understanding, according to Gadamer; Hans-Georg Gadamer, *Vérité et méthode. Les grandes lignes d'une herméneutique philosophique*, ed. Alain Badiou and Barbara Cassin, L'ordre philosophique (Paris: Seuil, 1996 [1960]), 298–312.
14 de Certeau, *La fable mystique II. XVIe-XVIIe siècle*, 166.

above about the biomedical and clinical discourse and its strong tendency to reduce the spiritual experience to self-development and wellbeing, other examples from the healthcare world amply demonstrate the language-related dimension of the spiritual experience. A survey of the literature and the general field shows that the philosophy of palliative care and associated concepts—total pain or suffering, comfort, relief, mitigation of pain—are used as facilitators in taking into account patients' spiritual experiences by doctors, nurses and other members of the care staff.[15] In other words, the language forged in the palliative care environment has a strong influence over the way in which caregivers view and speak about their patients' spiritual experience, and it is through the mediation of this vocabulary that spiritual experience takes form. At the same time, the vocabulary formats the way in which the caregivers pay attention to and identify what they call "the spiritual experience" for their patients. Similarly, in the scientific literature on nephrology, consideration for the spiritual experience is adjusted to match one of the main objectives of dialysis, which is its contribution to making patients persevere with their treatment.[16] Here, spirituality is understood as a possible support for perseverance with the technoscientific treatment for end-stage renal disease.

These two examples show convincingly that the language about spirituality used in a given community—here, in the literature on two specific care sectors—orients perceptions about what the spiritual experience during illness is. They also show that the spiritual experience is not fully formed before it is stated, but retains a degree of plasticity as it is moulded by language.

It is possible to object that a conception of spirituality like the one proposed by de Certeau leaves little room for the freedom, creativity and spontaneity generally associated with the spiritual experience by individuals in Western societies. However, we must not fall into the trap set by language. De Certeau's comments are not intended to form part of a philosophy of freedom or a sociology of creativity. In other words, he is not challenging the fundamental discourse on human freedom. On the other hand, he promotes the social dimension of the spiritual experience,[17] which may surprise some people in the present day, including many Christians for whom the spiritual experience, the ultimate zone of per-

---

15 Guy Jobin et al., "Spirituality, according to palliative caregivers. A systemic Analysis (Wie Spiritualität in Palliative Care verstanden wird. Eine Systemische Analyse," *Spiritual Care* 2, no. 1 (2013).
16 Guy Jobin, "La prise en compte de l'expérience spirituelle en soins palliatifs: un cas de mutation des représentations de la spiritualité," *Laval théologique et philosophique* 72, no. 3 (octobre 2016). Cf. also section 5.2.1 of chapter 5.
17 Sheldrake, *Explorations in Spirituality. History, Theology, dans Social Practice*, 118.

sonal freedom, can only be a purely personal experience. Nevertheless, besides identifying the language-related and social dimension of all spiritual discourses, de Certeau also points out another reality that is key to my argument: the fact that we never have direct access to the spiritual experience of others. Language sets a limit, and acts as a filter. It mediates between experience and any attempt to interpret it, including by the subject. The clear example of the "smokescreen" imposed by language is the case of apophatic theology which, paradoxically, uses words to describe the ineffable, with a clear and vivid awareness of the impassable gulf between what signifies and what is signified. Believers or theologians who want to talk about God using the apophatic style know, from the outset, that their discourse will always fall short of the reality they are attempting to understand or describe. Mystics are always acutely aware of this when they put their spiritual experience in writing, systematically, in the form of a story or poem.[18] Last, does the *Divine Comedy* not end with an avowal of ultimate incommunicability, when Dante contemplates God himself?[19]

In short, by taking into account the language-related dimension of the spiritual experience we can highlight the bias that affects any attempt to define the experience of or operationalize spirituality for pragmatic purposes, however laudable it may be, such as the effort made in the healthcare world to integrate patients' spiritual experiences as part of the clinical process.

7.2 Tradition

Although it is not explicitly addressed in the excerpt from *The Mystic Fable II*, the question of tradition is still present in passing in the idea of a language that exists before individuals and of a community that validates individual positions. Language and community are two vectors of tradition, because they convey nor-

---

18 Teresa of Avila wrote several books (*Autobiography, Book of Foundations*) that contain details about her spiritual experiences. John of the Cross used a hybrid poetical-systematical mode in *La montée du Carmel* and *Cantique spirituel*.

19 "Now my speech will fall further short, of what I remember, than a babe's, who still moistens his tongue at the breast. O how the words fall short, and how feeble compared with my conceiving! And they are such, compared to what I saw, that it is inadequate to call them merely feeble. Power, here, failed the deep imagining: but already my desire and will were rolled, like a wheel that is turned, equally, by the Love that moves the Sun and the other stars." Dante Alighieri, *La divine comédie: le paradis = [paradisio]: texte original*, trans. Jacqueline Risset (Paris: Flammarion, 1992), Canto XXXIII, verses 106–07; 21–23; 42–45.

mative content and are agents for its transmission.[20] Both the spiritual experience of a recognized mystic, and the spiritual experience of the man or woman in the street, are subject to the normative force of tradition, whether explicit or not.

This leads to a necessary conclusion. A spiritual discourse, of any kind, is always part of a tradition and, in addition, of a language tradition. There can be no spiritual discourse outside a tradition. This hermeneutic evidence also applies to contemporary spiritual discourses, even those that state that they are not anchored in any religious or lay tradition.

This "rule" that spiritual discourses are always anchored in tradition is also valid for biomedical and clinical language.[21] For example, the distinction between personal spirituality and collective religion, a central aspect as discussed above, derives from a modern tradition illustrated by Jean-Jacques Rousseau in his *Profession de foi du vicaire savoyard* [22] in which the philosopher presents a personal religion of the heart that he sets up in opposition to official dogmatic and authoritarian religion.[23] The theme of an individual religious experience that is truer and more authentic runs through modernity and forms the matrix for contemporary spiritual discourses. Here lies the paradox that I mentioned at the start of this chapter: the discourse that affirms the independence of the spiritual experience, as compared to the established traditions, is itself the product of a tradition. When the situation is analyzed, it is clear that the contemporary discourses have the fundamental anthropological characteristics of all human discourses.

The question raised by this observation is this: what is the status of this recent tradition of spiritual language compared to older religious and spiritual traditions, still present in the present-day cultural landscape? The fundamental statement of the modern spiritual tradition, namely that human beings are anthropologically spiritual, and culturally (or accidentally) religious,[24] carries a value judgment since, in this specific case, the universality ascribed to spiritual-

---

20 The word "tradition", from the Latin *"traditio"*, is used to designate two complementary realities: a process of transmission, and the content transmitted.
21 Jobin, *Des religions à la spiritualité. Une appropriation biomédicale du religieux dans l'hôpital*, 44–62.
22 Jean-Jacques Rousseau, *Profession de foi du vicaire savoyard*, folio essais (Paris: Gallimard, 1969[1762]).
23 Jobin, *Des religions à la spiritualité. Une appropriation biomédicale du religieux dans l'hôpital*, 45–51.
24 Jobin, *Des religions à la spiritualité. Une appropriation biomédicale du religieux dans l'hôpital*, 16.

ity appears to claim that the spiritual experience is superior to the religious experience. In this definition, what is considered to be universal has more value than what is cultural, and religion is seen as being a partial translation, within a given tradition, of the universal spiritual experience. Logically, this definition affirms the superiority of modern tradition over the religious traditions.

While avoiding the meanders of a relativist argument, it is important to state that there are no intrinsic reasons to support this aspect of the biomedical and clinical discourse about the spiritual experience during illness or, conversely, to place the discourse below the spiritual traditions that are part of a religious tradition. In other words, the biomedical and clinical discourse on spirituality is one spiritual language tradition among others, and is neither better nor worse than those that came before it. Factors that are extrinsic to the discourse explain its preponderance in the healthcare world, such as the social context of secularization, and the loss of credibility of the religious authorities and the traditions they represent. The question is to decide if these social, political and ecclesial factors are enough to assess the value of a spiritual tradition or religious tradition. The question carries its own answer. Without militancy or conviction, there is little chance of finding any criteria that will justify any claim that spirituality is superior to religious tradition.

We have seen how language and tradition are important for an anthropologically accurate understanding of the spiritual experience. We must now look in more depth at the role played by the third element: the group.

7.3 The group

It is possible to raise the objection that the idea of community of language underlying de Certeau's analysis applies only to the religious world and cannot take into account all the complexities and subtlety of the social and institutional dynamics that support contemporary spiritual discourses. Of course, in the world studied by de Certeau, the "community"—in this case, a Jesuit spiritual family drawing inspiration from 16th-century Spanish Carmelite mysticism—represents a group that, although it still exists, represents only one type of group among many others.

In the era of the "subjective turn,"[25] it appears that the notion of "network" is more useful to describe the configuration of the groups associated with contemporary schools of spiritual thought. From a sociological point of view, the no-

---

25 Heelas and Woodhead, *The spiritual revolution: why religion is giving way to spirituality,* 2–5.

tion of network reshuffles the habitual conceptual dichotomies: society/community, society/individual, community/individual. Sociologist of religions Raymond Lemieux presents the notion of "network" to report on belief in the present-day context. In his view, a network provides a better representation, at least conceptually, of the groups created by the current fascination with spiritual life. Some of these present-day practices are not regulated by communities. To illustrate the distinction he introduces, Lemieux contrasts the Christian belief of incarnation—regulated by the magisterium of the Catholic Church, a clearly identifiable authority in a community with clear and precise institutional boundaries—with the belief in reincarnation for which "there is no Church [...] or formal group controlling the conceptions and modes of dissemination of this belief among the new religious movements."[26] In this more diffuse environment, present-day spiritual discourses are subject to "reticular regulation,"[27] which operates using channels of communication based on contemporary means: books, film[28] and virtual (social) media, in other words reticular and, therefore, supra-community, media.[29]

However, networks still have normative force. This is why Lemieux talks about reticular regulation, even though the regulation involves plausibility and proposal rather than the community effect of a formal call for adherence to truth.[30] Although reticular regulation is not authoritarian in the same way as the Catholic magisterium, it is no less effective since it can effect a selection in the "set of available beliefs" to give precedence to particular specific beliefs or content. The same applies to the distancing/hierarchization of spirituality and religion, which has become the main way to understand the question of meaning today. This is also the case, in particular, of the lay or humanist traditions, a main element of which is the axiom that gives spirituality an anthropological status that is more fundamental than that of religion, as we saw above.

Even though social regulation of the spiritual experience appears to run through networks rather than traditional communities, it remains a genuine

---

26 Raymond Lemieux, "La dialectique de la communauté et du réseau dans le champ religieux," in *Communautés et socialités Formes et force du lien social dans la modernité tardive*, ed. Francine Saillant and Éric Gagnon (Montréal: Liber, 2005): 81.
27 Lemieux, "La dialectique de la communauté et du réseau dans le champ religieux": 81.
28 Including the movies *Pay It Forward*, 2000 and *Eat, Pray, Love*, 2010.
29 Obviously, since the article by Lemieux was written, the Catholic Church, for example, uses network-like methods in its communication strategies. However, they are still subject to a form of community regulation embodied in the magisterium.
30 Lemieux, "La dialectique de la communauté et du réseau dans le champ religieux": 82.

form of regulation. It therefore involves a language and a group, whatever its form and, last, a tradition, even if recently founded.

These few comments on spiritual anthropology are made to show that the biomedical and clinical language cannot escape the same determining factors as any discourse on the spiritual experience, and is subject to the same hermeneutic constraints as other attempts to relate experience using language. It possesses the same paradoxical power of revelation and occultation of human experience, since it is merely one of many different forms of mediation.

7.4 The "materiality" of spiritual life

In addition to the anthropologically inescapable elements of language, tradition and group, a fourth issue arises when setting the markers of the spiritual experience: the nature of the spiritual experience during illness.

As we have seen, the new openness to spirituality in the clinical environment occurred, partly, thanks to the introduction of a new medical model, the bio-psycho-social approach.[31] The model, adopted and implemented in several care sectors (palliative care, oncology, psychiatry, etc.), promoted interdisciplinary responsibility for each patient. In the wake of the transforming model proposed by Engel, physician and theologian Daniel P. Sulmasy suggested adding spirituality to the model's other categories,[32] and care teams were asked to pay attention to the repercussions of illness in the four dimensions proposed and justified by the model. This model is based on philosophical anthropology, as explained by Sulmasy in an article published in 2002. The patient is viewed as the meeting-point of four complementary and interwoven relationships: the physical relationships of body parts, mind-body relationships (which constitute the person), the relationship with the interpersonal environment, and the relationship with the transcendent. Spirituality is present especially in the three last types of relationship: body/mind, person/others, and person/transcendence.

We have also seen how, from the emergence of palliative care, the concept of total pain could include the dying person's spiritual experience.

---

31 Chapter 4, section 4.3.
32 Daniel P. Sulmasy, *The Rebirth of the Clinic. An Introduction to Spirituality in Health Care* (Washington, D.C.: Georgetown University Press, 2007); Daniel P. Sulmasy, "A biopsychosocial-spiritual model for the care of patients at the end of life," *Gerontologist* 42 Spec No 3 (2002); Alan B. Astrow, Christina M. Puchalski, and Daniel P. Sulmasy, "Religion, spirituality, and health care: social, ethical, and practical considerations," *Am J Med* 110, no. 4 (2001).

These developments, and others, helped "embody" (in both the figurative and literal meanings) a "material" representation of spirituality. In the clinical language, spirituality is not only something that is heard,[33] but also "something" that is revealed through its effects, manifestations, influence over the body, personality, etc. In other words, this representation of spiritual life refers back to the image of a "thing", which is of course precious, unique, fundamental and individual to each person, but is also a "thing" that can be active, by influencing other dimensions of the person, or passive, by enduring the impacts of illness. This is where the expression "spiritual dimension" takes on more density and becomes a locatable reality, and even one that can be manipulated through work on the body or psyche or, inversely, is able to work on the body and psyche. The spiritual dimension of human beings, referred to as the "spirit" in the literature, is located at the intersection of the psychic and the somatic.

For anyone who knows a little about history, the process I describe above bears a close resemblance to something that happened at a key moment in the birth of Western medicine. When the contemporary discourse on the spirit is compared to the Christian discourse on the soul, we can see the result of a process that is similar to what happened to illness in the Hippocratic medical tradition. The Copernican revolution brought about by Hippocrates—if we can be excused this anachronism!—was to return the causes of illness and health to Earth.[34] They no longer depended on the arbitrary actions of the gods, or on the ability of specific human intermediaries to deflect divine wishes through sacrifices or worship-based exercises. Thanks to Hippocrates and his disciples, sickness and health were related, respectively, to a bad or good physiological balance, in the well-known doctrine of the four humours. The Hippocratic school located the origin of sickness and health in the body, its operations and its reactions to the environment. In technical terms, this is referred to as the intramondanization of the causes of sickness and health, which are located in the world as we know it.

The "locating" of spirituality within human beings reflects a similar displacement. The soul—spiritual and immaterial—is no longer the locus of spirituality, as the link between an individual and God. In the humanist/lay conception of spirituality, the spirit, the psychic dimension of each person and one that is not necessarily linked to any form of transcendence, is the locus of spirituality.

---

33 Maxime Allard, "De la possibilité d'entendre du 'spirituel' en fin de vie," in *Spiritualités et biomédecine Enjeux d'une intégration*, ed. Guy Jobin, Jean-Marc Charron, and Michel Nyabenda (Québec: Presses de l'Université Laval, 2013).

34 Jobin, *Des religions à la spiritualité. Une appropriation biomédicale du religieux dans l'hôpital*, 84–86.

Spirituality is brought "back to Earth", like the Hippocratic representation of sickness. Spirituality has become, within the body, a "place" or "dimension"—both terms with spatial connotations—from which emanations (feelings, convictions, beliefs, values, desires, etc.) that can be mobilized during times of illness. The intramondanization of spirituality is combined, here, with a form of reification, which makes spiritual life a "thing". The recent tendency to represent spirituality in this way is clearly promoted by research. For example, research into the neurocognitive foundations for the spiritual experience have been published in several different specialized neuroscience journals.[35] In addition, a research area, known by the name of neurotheology, is attempting to demonstrate the biological foundations for belief and faith[36] and for the spiritual experience during an epileptic seizure.[37] The brain, and its complex architecture and operations, are the key targets for this search for material evidence of spiritual life in human beings.

It must be admitted that neurotheology and the use of imaging to find the biological foundations of spirituality are based on a radical conception of the materiality of spiritual life. They are, for now, the most obvious examples. The reification of spiritual life is not, however, limited to these extreme manifesta-

---

35 Joseph M. Barnby et al., "How similar are the changes in neural activity resulting from mindfulness practice in contrast to spiritual practice?," *Conscious Cogn* 36 (2015); Cristiano Crescentini et al., "Virtual lesions of the inferior parietal cortex induce fast changes of implicit religiousness/spirituality," *Cortex* 54 (2014); Anders Hougaard et al., "Evidence of a Christmas spirit network in the brain: functional MRI study," *Bmj* 351 (2015); Jeong-H. Kim et al., "Self-transcendence trait and its relationship with in vivo serotonin transporter availability in brainstem raphe nuclei: An ultra-high resolution PET-MRI study," *Brain Res* 1629 (2015); Rüdiger J. Seitz, Raymond F. Paloutzian, and Hans-Ferdinand Angel, "Processes of believing: Where do they come from? What are they good for?," *F1000Res* 5 (2016); Mahsa Vaghefi et al., "Spirituality and brain waves," *J Med Eng Technol* 39, no. 2 (2015); Michiel van Elk and André Aleman, "Brain mechanisms in religion and spirituality: An integrative predictive processing framework," *Neurosci Biobehav Rev* 73 (2017).
36 Eugene G. D'Aquili and Andrew B. Newberg, *The mystical mind: probing the biology of religious experience* (Minneapolis, MN: Fortress Press, 1999); Andrew B. Newberg, *Principles of neurotheology* (Farnham, Surrey, England: Ashgate Pub, 2010); Andrew B. Newberg, Eugene G. D'Aquili, and Vince Rause, *Why God won't go away: brain science and the biology of belief*, 1st ed. (New York: Ballantine Books, 2001); Andrew B. Newberg, Eugene G. D'Aquili, and Vince Rause, *Pourquoi "Dieu" ne disparaîtra pas: quand la science explique la religion* (Vannes: Sully, 2003); Andrew B. Newberg and Mark Robert Waldman, *Why we believe what we believe: uncovering our biological need for meaning, spirituality, and truth* (New York: Free Press, 2006); Andre B. Newberg and Mark Robert Waldman, *Words can change your brain: 12 conversation strategies to build trust, resolve conflict, and increase intimacy* (New York: Plume, 2013).
37 Niall McCrae and Rob Whitley, "Exaltation in Temporal Lobe Epilepsy: Neuropsychiatric Symptom or Portal to the Divine?," *Journal of Medical Humanities* 35, no. 3 (2014).

tions. In a more benign, but still significant, way, spiritual assessment question-naires[38] reflect the same goal of measuring the spiritual experience in order to act on its determinants, when the person is considered to be in spiritual distress.

The fact remains that this trend towards an "intramondane" interpretation of the spiritual experience, which can go as far as a materialistic interpretation, is a clear trend in biomedical and clinical thought.

7.5 Conclusion to chapter seven

Our personal spiritual experience cannot escape from the constraints of history and culture. This does not mean that it is completely determined by the contin-gencies inherent in human life, but their historicity must certainly be taken into account. By taking the language-related, traditional and "community" character of the spiritual experience seriously, it becomes possible to consider it outside the reductive framework of universalizing thought. In the end, the singularity of the spiritual experience can only gain from this. It may appear paradoxical to link the traditional and "community" character of the spiritual experience to its singularity, but this apparent paradox is resolved once the singular person-al experience is placed within the language tradition that supports it. In this way, the temptation to apply a universal framework of interpretation will, in principle, be avoided.

---

38 Discussed in chapter 5, section 5.1.2.

8 The spiritual experience as a response to an event

Is there a way to look at the spiritual experience that does not involve making it a strictly psychic dimension of individual human beings? Can it also be examined in terms of the fundamental anthropological characteristics presented in the preceding chapter? At the same time, is it possible to imagine an articulation between spirituality and ethics without relying on the sapiential form of theological thought? I believe that a promising avenue for answering these questions, at least in part, lies in the proposals made by philosopher and theologian John D. Caputo concerning the theology of the event. This theological proposition is not primarily concerned with spirituality, but provides input for a discussion of tradition, religious language, spiritual language, and the relationship that may be formed between two or more spiritual traditions. My hypothesis is that the work of Caputo provides enough material to address the questions outlined above. But before going any further in this reflection on the spiritual experience using the work of Caputo, I should say a few words about the contribution made by theology to a reflective understanding of the "spiritual question" today.

8.1 Contribution of the theological discourse to present-day discussions of spirituality

Is it really necessary to introduce a theological discourse into contemporary conversations about the spiritual experience? This is not simply a rhetorical question. As we have seen, the link between religious experience—and consequentially, the discipline of theology which "studies" it—and spiritual experience is not a foregone conclusion in contemporary culture. Let us not forget that theology is, ideally, a process that seeks to describe the faith experience of a community of belief, based on its founding documents and its rites, in short by the representations of humanity contained in the documents and rites, which are dogmatic and theological constructs that attempt to set the boundaries of what the community considers to be an authentic faith experience. After all, theology, or faith seeking understanding (*fides quaerens intellectum*, in the words of Anselm of Canterbury), is a "sectorial" discourse whose relevance is limited by the boundaries of the community of faith that produces it. What could it possibly have to say about the spiritual paths followed by the contemporary population, chosen specifically because they remain at a distance from the fields covered,

https://doi.org/10.1515/9783110638950-009

respectively, by the traditional religions?[1] In these conditions, how can the theological discourse be included in present-day discussions about the spiritual experience? And more specifically, how can it form part of the interdisciplinary conversation about the spiritual experience taking place in the healthcare world?

These questions are relevant and valid for a theological discourse that seeks to understand faith within a community of believers. This is an important, but not the only function of theology, since its target audience is also society.[2] Presenting the act of faith and the content of faith to citizens both with and without a religious or spiritual affiliation is one of the tasks of theology. This theological endeavour does not aim to convert the population or ensure a return to the Church/State relationship that prevailed in the time of Christianity. In fact, the role of theology here is to present the internal coherence of the act of faith (and its content) and to reflect on the contribution made by believers to building a shared world that is habitable for all. In the present case, the issue is to question biomedical and clinical representations and practices from a theological point of view.

The approach taken here is what I call a "confrontation of traditions", which can be expressed as a question: what would result from a confrontation between the modern tradition of spirituality—which forms the basis for the biomedical and clinical discourse on the matter—and the long tradition of reflection and support practices for the spiritual experience, which are so widespread in Christianity?

What does the word "confrontation" mean in this context? It is neither a fusion of the traditions nor a search for a common denominator. Neither is it an attempt to subordinate one tradition to the other, one example of which is the contemporary discourse that makes spirituality a concept that incorporates religion, giving a positive value to spirituality and a negative value to religion.

The objective of the confrontation is for the traditions to shed light on each other, without looking for a third option to act as an interface between them or

1 See the description given by Stolz et al. of alternative spirituality or religiosity completed detached from traditional religion: Stolz et al., *Religion et spiritualité à l'ère de l'ego: profils de l'institutionnel, de l'alternatif, du distancié et du séculier [Religion and spirituality in the era of the ego. Institutional, alternative, distancing and secular profiles]*, 115–21. Cf. also Robert C. Fuller, *Spiritual, but not religious understanding unchurched America*, (Oxford: Oxford University Press, 2001), http://dx.doi.org/10.1093/0195146808.001.0001.; Heelas and Woodhead, *The spiritual revolution: why religion is giving way to spirituality*; Phil Zuckerman, *Faith no more: why people reject religion* (New York: Oxford University Press, 2012).
2 David Tracy, *The analogical imagination: Christian theology and the culture of pluralism* (New York: Crossroad, 1981).

bring them together. With this safeguard in place, can the traditions question each other about their *a priori* positions, their interpretational frameworks and their plans for action? Can Christianity, with its long experience of reflections and practices in connection with the spiritual experience, highlight some of the traps awaiting the biomedical and clinical discourse on spirituality?

How should this research aim be implemented and directed? I propose an approach based on the work of theologian John Caputo, which provides a partial response to the questions posed in the introduction to this chapter. This partial exploration of the work of Caputo may seem arduous to readers who are not familiar with theology and philosophy, both of which are called into play by Caputo.

I have planned the chapter as follows. The first section (8.2.) offers a brief overview of the characteristics of theology of the event. This is followed by a methodological explanation (8.3.) that aims to report on the "approach" of theology of the event. Then, I offer a reflection on the spiritual experience using theology of the event. (8.4.) It is followed by some thoughts on the articulation between ethics and spirituality (8.5.) A few words on spirituality and the event concludes this exploration (8.6.)

8.2 Theology of the event

John Caputo is a US intellectual who is both a philosopher of religion and theologian, and a deconstructionist influenced by the work of French philosopher Jacques Derrida. Derrida remains a constant reference for Caputo, who presents his work in a constant dialogue with other key names in contemporary philosophy, including Emmanuel Levinas in particular, Alain Badiou and Jean-François Lyotard, and theologians in the Western tradition such as Augustine and Pierre Damien. He is also an interpreter of biblical texts, which provide a primary methodological source for his reflection. In short, Caputo, as a good post-modernist, is an example of theoretical eclecticism.

He describes his theological contributions as weak theology[3] or radical theology, resulting from "short circuits". This designates the mobilization of argumentative strategies that bring together authors who, at first sight, are not intellectually related. One clear example of this type of short circuit in the work of

---

3 Recalling the "weak thought" proposed by Gianni Vattimo.

Caputo is the confrontation between the works of the Apostle Paul and Jacques Derrida—the short circuit involves reading Paul through the work of Derrida.[4]

Caputo's approach is articulated around the thesis "that the name of God is an event, or rather that it *harbors* an event, and that theology is the hermeneutics of that event, its task being to release what is happening in that name, to set it free, to give it its own head, and thereby to head off the forces that would prevent this event."[5] Caputo distances himself from a metaphysical and affirmative style of theology that formulates a positive discourse on the ontological nature of God, a traditional style that he describes as "strong theology" in which "God is the highest being in the order of presence (overseeing and insuring the presence of order), who presides over the order of being and manifestations."[6] However, Caputo does not reject the Trinity, but does reject the idea of dealing with the question of God using ontological and metaphysical terms inherited from the philosophical tradition of Antiquity, which makes God a being above all others; a being with no limits on his power and will; the first unmoved mover;[7] etc. At the same time, he criticizes any form of theology structured around a theory of two worlds, including the emblematic work of Saint Augustine (354–430 CE).[8] According to Augustine, there exist two worlds that he names respectively Earthly City and City of God, built on two different and opposing principles: "Accordingly, two cities have been formed by two loves: the earthly by the love of self, even to the contempt of God; the heavenly by the love of God, even to the contempt of self."[9] Caputo associates this strong theology with metaphysical thought, in particular when it distinguishes between the human world and the supernatural world.

The theology of the event proposed by Caputo is destabilizing for anyone seeking to mobilize the traditional modes of theological thought. His description proceeds negatively[10] highlighting what the event is not.

---

4 John D. Caputo, *The Weakness of God. A Theology of the Event*, ed. Merod Westhal, Indiana Series in the Philosophy of Religion (Bloomington: Indiana University Press, 2006), 12–13.
5 Caputo, *The Weakness of God. A Theology of the Event*, 2.
6 Caputo, *The Weakness of God. A Theology of the Event*, 8–9.
7 An expression inherited from Aristotle's philosophy.
8 John D. Caputo, *The Insistence of God. A Theology of Perhaps*, ed. Merod Westhal, Indiana Series in the Philosophy of Religion (Bloomington: Indiana University Press, 2013), 64–65; 99–101.
9 Augustine, *The City of God*, books XIV, XXVIII.
10 Here, the weak theology proposed by Caputo resembles the apophatic style of theology, even if Caputo considers apophatism to be a strong (but silent) theology: Caputo, *The Weakness of God. A Theology of the Event*, 36.

8.2.1 The event is "uncontainable"

The event is not a thing that can be circumscribed using a proper or common noun, a concept or an idea. The event is not limited by a semantic field. Caputo, describing himself as a "nominalist"[11] states that an event overflows the noun that hosts it. The name of an event (God, democracy, love, the Kingdom of God, justice, truth, sickness, death, etc.) is only a partial translation and actualization of the event it hosts. This is why other names can be associated with the event, with no ill effect. This initial characteristic of weak theology already points to a key element of Caputo's approach: the gap between what is designated by language, and the words we use in attempting to designate it. This gap cannot be filled. No language allows us to fully and completely understand the event.

8.2.2 The event cannot be seized by traditional metaphysical thought

Caputo repeats unceasingly: there is no metaphysical link between the name and the event.[12] This characteristic is closely connected to the "uncontainability" of the event in a name. In Caputo's view, the source of this unfillable gap is the fact that the event is not in the realm of being. The event is a call. In fact, the source of the call is intangible. This precision, which marks a change from the traditional perspective, is crucial. The call is a trace, in other words a mark or clue of what is no longer there. The call is not God, it is the event hosted by the word "God" that is everything except being. Radical, or weak, theology does not attempt to describe the being of God; it focuses only on what remains of his passage, namely the trace in the form of a call. In the technical language of theology, we can say that weak theology is not an ontology; instead, it is a hermeneutic of the trace,[13] in other words it seeks to interpret the call contained in the word "God". The following sections add some details to the resulting interpretative gesture.

---

11 Caputo, *The Weakness of God. A Theology of the Event*, 3.
12 This repetition is necessary, since the invitation to think about God otherwise than through historically-inherited categories is often heard, but seldom understood in the full depth of its radicalness.
13 Caputo, *The Insistence of God. A Theology of Perhaps*, 106.

8.2.3 Excess

An event occurs independently of me, of us. It comes towards us. The event is an eruption that disturbs our daily routine. It is an excess for us and our everyday lives. This is why Caputo states that an event is also an advent. Eruption, excess, overflowing: the event has all the characteristics of something situated beyond economy, exchange and transaction. The event is more than give-and-take or a simple equivalence. In fact, because of its excessive dimension,[14] the event is a gift with no return, a gift for which there is no possible response or equivalent counter-gift. The event upsets the expectation of a return, which seems so "natural" for a person living in a world where commercial logic prevails.

In corollary with excess, the event requires a horizon of expectations, but not to force compliance, as if new wine could be put into old wineskins without bursting them! Instead, the horizon of expectations designates what will be invested, upset and torn by the paradoxically strong weak force, destabilizing and unusual, of the event. The event must upset something else and move it. The disturbances caused by the event make it recognizable, the disturbances caused by the eruption of that which presents itself as the other aspect of what was expected. One example of destabilization in daily life is love at first sight, which is unplanned and involves an eruption of a complex set of feelings, and is an emotional and human experience that happens without notice. The birth of a child and the experience of parenthood is an excess, an event, that takes place over the long term and changes a life.

8.2.4 The event as a promise

In addition to its excessive nature, the event is a promise to be kept, a call that requires a response, a prayer to be granted, a hope to be realized. In short, the event is always fragile and precarious, since it requires a response if its effects are to be felt in an individual and collective life. The event is, in fact, at the mercy of the person who hears its call. What is to come, the possibility that the promise will be realized, depends on a response, a form of responsibility on the part of the hearers of the call, in other words you and me. However, there are obstacles on the path: interference may prevent the call from being heard, or there may be a form of deafness, whether voluntary or not, to the

---

14 Obviously, excess appears only in the eyes of those who calculate, weight, or look for equivalency...

call. This occurs, for example, when a common or proper noun no longer attracts interest in the event it hosts. For example, the name of "God" does not resonate in the same way in a secular society as it does in a society where there is a state religion.

In addition, the event is not necessarily a happy one. It may be negative. Once again, the name of "God" is the example given by Caputo. The history of the use of this name bears witness to both good and bad. "God" is a high-risk word.

> The fluctuation between the sacrifice of others to my will and the sacrifice of my will in the service of others is built into the name (of) "God" in just the same way the best and the worst are built into other high-velocity words like justice and democracy, truth and love. The higher the velocity at which these words speed along, the higher the stakes for good and evil. The name (of) "God" calls forth the best and the worst. It is the riskiest name we know and you cannot simply decontaminate it of it undecidability.[15]

8.2.5 Time

An event takes place in time, but in *kairos* rather than in chronological time, using the classical distinction between *chronos* and *kairos*.[16] *Chronos* designates unqualified time that runs without interruption, smoothly, in other words time that is simply duration. It is time as measured by a watch. *Kairos* is the time of opportunity, of destiny, of meaning, the time that appears dense, full of meaning, in which every moment counts. *Kairos* is an eruption of something that appears to come from elsewhere, a "break" in a banal routine, and even a breach in the uniform movement of time. In short, the event is something that we do not see coming; it is what occurs in what is happening or, even more succinctly, what insists in what exists.

8.2.6 Desire

Last, the event is a desire that lies well beyond earthly desires—prestige, fame, fortune, etc.—and beyond "celestial" desires such as salvation. An event goes beyond these first-order desires. The desire created by the event is a desire that has no name, the desire of a promise that has no other visage than what is to come, the visage of a promise. So, "what we desire is not what it is but what it promises

---

15 Caputo, *The Insistence of God. A Theology of Perhaps*, 108.
16 The Greek words *kairos* and *chronos* designate two ways of experiencing time.

to be, or rather what is being promised in the desire. First-order desire is directed at something formed and constituted, while a desire beyond desire is elicitated by the event that has been contracted into the first-order object of desire."[17] The desire beyond desire has not object. Caputo uses the French expression of "je ne sais quoi" to designate this object that is not an object, the desire of je-ne-sais-quoi. In fact, the dynamics of desire beyond desire require a form of passivity from the desirer, the corollary of the initiative taken by the event or call.

8.3 Methodological explanation

I have just outlined some of the characteristics of the "weak" or "radical" theology proposed by John Caputo. His description of theology of the event,[18] in 2006, was followed by a methodological explanation in 2013, in what Caputo called "theology of perhaps."[19] This theological exploration of the event hidden in the name (of) "God" began with the starting-point of the denominational religious traditions, which Caputo considers to be responses that demonstrate the existence, that make concrete, the insistent call that both precedes and constitutes them. The theological traditions developed during the historical deployment of Christianity and the meeting of several cultures, are an example of a response to the call contained in the name (of) "God".

The methodological issue presented by Caputo is to trace and expose the event hidden at the heart of these denominational theologies. The theology of the event addresses the task using the theologies themselves, considered as reflective discourses about the beliefs and practices of a community or group. It is the reflective effort, which seeks to make the faith experience intelligible, that is the primary project of radical theology, and not beliefs and practices as such.

The event will be heard within the limits set by a traditional discourse. Caputo repeats, in his own way, the importance of traditions and language which, in his eyes, are traces of past responses, of effects, or of traces of the trace. In pursuit of this goal, radical theology deploys two approaches: displacement and affirmation, which I will examine in turn.

---

17 Caputo, *The Insistence of God. A Theology of Perhaps*, 84.
18 Several expressions are used to describe this specific form of theology as applied by Caputo: theology of perhaps, circumfessional theology, non-foundational theology, parasitic theology compared to denominational theologies, etc. The multiplicity of possible names refers back to Caputo's own nominalism, which highlights the impossibility of enclosing the event in a concept or single name.
19 Caputo, *The Insistence of God. A Theology of Perhaps*.

8.3.1 Displacement

Displacement haunts the denominational theologies in the form of the expression "perhaps", which destabilizes the posture that makes tradition the site of ultimate truth and a sure support for the construction of the believer's identity. Adding the expression "perhaps" to theological propositions highlights the inevitable historical and contingent nature of all theological traditions. The attachment of "perhaps" to a theological tradition results, in fact, from a strong sensitivity to the hermeneutic question and the historical development of the ecclesial traditions of faith and practice. The tradition—and by extension all traditions—are understood as a historical product, in other words as the accumulation of cognitive, practical, aesthetic, and ethical elements that reflect a vision of the world, organized as a whole that is intended to be coherent. This historical nature of a tradition does not mean that it is necessarily without relevance for an adherent. By emphasizing the historical nature of the tradition, Caputo insists that it is a located, contextual and temporal response to the event that it carries within in.

If contingent traditions are displaced by the event, it is because there is a gap that structures the relationship between the call and the tradition, which Caputo describes using the idea of chiasma. A chiasma is the intertwining of the call and the response, of that which insists (the call coming from the name (of) "God") and that which exists (denominational theology). Intertwining is not merging. The applicable image here is the weaving of a rope or cable from separate strands. The end result is a cable, and not a thicker strand made up of all the others. Intertwining means that a gap is maintained, however small, between the strands. The distance between the call and the response cannot be crossed, meaning that the call will always exceed the traditions that respond. Because of the basic uncertainty and undecidability it engenders, the "perhaps" blocks any attempt to identify the tradition completely with the call.

In addition, the "perhaps" projects the image that a tradition is never a definitive response. It is, at best, a penultimate word, leaving us waiting for the last word. Tradition is, at best, a partial response to the call. In short, the "perhaps" has the power to destabilize certainties and displace outside positions of absolute knowledge. Caputo adds that the destabilizing effect is not limited to traditions, since its effects can be felt by individuals.

The "perhaps" can also apply to personal adherence to a belief group. It shows the personal profession of faith in a new light, within a given denominational tradition. There is a (large) measure of chance in personal adherence to a denominational tradition: the chance of a person's place of birth and host culture, the chance of encounters during the socialization process, the chance of significant moments in the *kaïros*, in short, the chance of each personal and social pathway. Rather than ascribing a biographical journey to a plan designed by an other-worldly entity—such as a personal destiny decided by God—Caputo ascribes it to chance. His goal is not to make believers insecure or anxious, or to doubt the sincerity of their adherence. Rather, it is to point out that an individual's religious path varies depending on the spiritual/religious "ecosystem" of a given society. As a result, many Catholics are only Catholic because of the place and time of their birth, "perhaps".

The displacement induced by this "perhaps" therefore occurs on two levels: the level of tradition, and the level of the person.

One immediate question concerns Caputo's claim that radical theology is theological. How does it differ from historical criticism, sociological criticism or ideological criticism, in short from the discourses and analytical approaches that identify mechanisms for the conditioning of minds and individual and social behaviour? An exploration of the biblical roots of radical theology can answer this question and learn more about displacement, as presented by radical theology.

Caputo bases his reflection on the first letter to the Corinthians, more specifically the passage that reveals Paul's belief, concording with the expectations of the Christians he is addressing, in Christ's imminent return.[20] The belief has concrete implications for the lives of adherents. Paul instructs Christians to maintain their station in life, but without becoming attached to it. For example, he does not ask married people to end their marriage. Instead, he asks them, in light of the imminence of Christ's return and the resulting radical change in the world, to turn to what is coming without neglecting what already is. Marriage and celibacy, which he also gives as an example, are good ways to live for a Christian. They must be maintained, in the knowledge that they are transitory and do not, in themselves, bring salvation. He invites his readers to keep the promises they have made, but without letting themselves be "submerged" by the form or state of their lives. This example of a practical Christian life is transposed by Caputo to describe how to adhere to a tradition: adhering to it but without being submerged by it; forming part of it, but without making it the ultimate and definitive answer to the call heard. Like the gap created by the wait for Christ's return between a believer and his or her state of life, Caputo calls on

---

[20] In the King James version: "But this I say, brethren, the time is short: it remaineth, that both they that have wives be as though they had none; And they that weep, as though they wept not; and they that rejoice, as though they rejoiced not; and they that buy, as though they possessed not; And they that use this world, as not abusing it: for the fashion of this world passeth away.", 1Cor 7:29 – 31.

us to adhere to a tradition without becoming attached to its historical and social contingencies, while remaining open to the awaited event. This involves distinguishing between faith and belief—faith being related to a call, while belief is related to tradition.

This attitude dissociates the historical/contingent nature of traditions from the event that issues a call through a tradition. Caputo describes this as follows: "the call of the event subjects the call of the mundane confessional vocation to recall; one inhabits the belief as if not, weakening the belief in order to release the event. We weaken the intimidating prestige and enormous power of belief in order to release the pressure exerted by the soft voice of the event of faith [...]. [w] e suspend the mundane circumstances of "belief" in order to release the event of "faith"."[21] Everything happens as though the beliefs filled all spaces and gaps, and aimed to fix the tradition once and for all. Denouncing the overshadowing of faith by belief amounts to establishing the conditions needed for vigilance and the expectation of the event that is to come.

8.3.2 Affirmation

The second operational mode of radical theology is called "affirmation" by Caputo. It is closely linked to the destabilizing power of "perhaps". What is "affirmed" is not a new response to the call, since such a response would come under the responsibility of denominational theology. The "content" of the affirmation is to renew a "faith" in the destabilizing capacity of the event, in the questioning of first-order evidence, and in whatever upsets shared beliefs which, by definition or because of habit, are not discussed. Affirmation, too, is presented as a weak theology, like a phantom or spectre that haunts theology, "with a quiet but overwhelming unease over the insufficiency of their categories and of every project of objectification."[22] It is an affirmation of the vigilance that must be part of every theological project, a vigilance about the inevitable gap between the theological discourse and the call it seeks to answer.

Like apophatic theology and analogy, throughout the history of Christian theology,[23] Caputo's radical theology highlights the humility required for theological work. However, the difference between them and radical theology lies

---

21 Caputo, *The Insistence of God. A Theology of Perhaps*, 79.
22 Caputo, *The Insistence of God. A Theology of Perhaps*, 82.
23 Without going into the technical theological details, I should mention that apophatic theology and analogy are two forms of discourse that emerged as part of the Christian theological effort.

in the fact that the gap named is not ontological in nature. The gap lies else-where... it is what separates the insistence of a call from the existence of a tra-dition.

In conclusion to this brief exploration of Caputo's proposal, it is important to mention that radical theology emphasizes what the call achieves within denom-inational theologies: it calls on the faith community to answer the call through belief and practice; it invites theologians to examine the life of belief reflexively to seek its intelligence and coherence; it continually wields its weak strength of destabilization; it quietly denounces all the intellectual and dogmatic sclerosis of tradition, while sowing the concern of a "perhaps" over the rightness of the theological discourse about its "objects" of predilection.

The theoretical framework that structures radical theology applies, of course, to all forms of tradition. As I mentioned, after Caputo, the words "jus-tice", "democracy", "truth" and "love" harbour events, make calls and generate beliefs, practices and discourses that are, in fact, traditions. The call-tradition dy-namic is therefore not exclusive to the world of religion and theological reflec-tion. We can use this observation to shed more light on the delicate question of the way language traditions can influence the spiritual experience during ill-ness.

8.4 The event and the spiritual experience

We can now begin to think about the spiritual experience in light of the theory of the event and of radical theology, while being careful to avoid a fundamental error, the error of identification. It is only too tempting to attempt to equate the event with the spiritual experience. This would, however, be an error be-cause, as I have pointed out several times and in particular in the previous chap-ter, the spiritual experience is a phenomenon of language and tradition. The spi-ritual experience is dependent; it relies on a tradition of language to exist, and the language precedes the subject. It would be an error of category to think of the spiritual and religious experience as being identical to that which calls. In fact, the spiritual experience is what exists; it is the trace of an insistence. It is not the insistence itself.

Based on this fact, the elucidation of the spiritual experience I propose here is articulated around two axes, which I have called the axis of contextualization and the axis of alterity.

8.4.1 The axis of contextualization

Radical theology and the theory of the event on which it is based highlight the situated and contextual nature of the spiritual experience. At this level Caputo agrees with the conclusions of Michel de Certeau about the language-based and traditional nature of every spiritual experience.[24] The (individual or collective) spiritual experience occurs within a language tradition. By stating that the answer to the call is always contextual, Caputo reiterates the inescapable mediation performed by language and tradition.

The theory of the event highlights three crucial aspects of the spiritual experience and the traditions that embody it.

First, I have already discussed the implicit hierarchical relationship between spirituality and religion in the biomedical and clinical discourse[25] and stated that there are no criteria intrinsic to the traditions that support this vision. The theory of the event strengthens our reflection on the basic equality of the traditions of language, since they are situated, contextual responses to the call that haunts them. To the calls embodied in the words "God", "justice", "truth", etc., we can add the word "spirituality" in its lay sense.

Second, and following on from my first comment, the equality of status of the traditions of language does not mean that they can be reduced each to the other. Nothing requires the call to be the same in all the traditions. For example, it is clear that the call that underlies the western traditions of the discourse on justice differ from those whose "object" is love. The two words cannot, in addition, be reduced one in the other, since love is driven by a logic of giving and overabundance, while justice relies on a logic of equivalence.[26] This irreducibility is valid, as we have seen, for the traditions of spiritual and religious language.

Third, Caputo carefully avoids formulating any universalisms in his theory. He does not refer to "the" religion, but to denominational theological traditions. Just as the words "democracy" or "republic" evoke a plurality of traditions of thought and discourse, the word "spirituality" does not refer to a single phenomenon, but to a multitude of traditions of language. Epistemologically speaking, the search for the universal is a search for a concept that would embody all spiritual experiences. However, Caputo is wary of any concept that would embody all experiences or consist of one ultimate and insurmountable explanation of the phenomena, and also of any concept that would transcend the traditions and

---

24 Cf. chapter 7, section 7.1
25 Chapter 7, section 7.2.
26 Paul Ricœur, *Amour et justice* (Paris: Éditions Points, 2008).

games of language to fix the metaphysical reality of what is described.[27] Because Caputo's proposal is made within radical phenomenology and hermeneutics, his prudence approach to general judgments and respect for traditions and languages comes as no surprise.

By emphasizing the contextual aspect of the spiritual experience, Caputo's theory draws attention to its eminently contingent nature. Spiritual life, as experienced by human beings, is intimately linked to a given time and culture. This language-based and traditional status gives the spiritual experience—and also the religious experience—a precise place in the insistence-existence chiasm, on the same side as the human answer to the call.

The contingent nature of the spiritual experience also emphasizes the extent of its "fragility". The call resounds with the full force of its supplication and may result—but with no assurance of success—in a response by individual believers or communities of believers. The spiritual experience unfolds over time, in space and in the culture of individuals and groups. There is therefore no universal spiritual experience. The fact that these contingent experiences are present across many different cultures and epochs does not indicate that they are all equal and share the same characteristics. Since a growing number of people in the West describe themselves as neither spiritual nor religious, there is scope to question the universality of the spiritual experience as expounded in contemporary clinical theories.[28] The only answers are situated and contextual. History is full of such answers, which have then become institutionalized, and Netherlands theologian Kees Waaijman has divided into three groups the spiritual experiences that give rise to institutions: lay spiritualities, schools of spirituality, and spiritualities that underlie movements on the margins of power structures.[29]

---

27 Caputo's wariness is tangible in his technical discussion of the notion of concept in Hegel's philosophy (cf. Caputo, *The Insistence of God. A Theology of Perhaps*, 87–116. Chapter 5: "Two Types of Continental Philosophy of Religion"). He invokes headless Hegelianism. Without going into this discussion in detail, Caputo considers himself to be a heretical Hegelian who sees religion as a *Vorstellung*, as a representation that must be addressed poetically, rather than as a *Begriff*, a strictly rational and logical concept.

28 The work of Jörg Stoltz, cited above, shows the trend in Switzerland towards the disaffiliation of individuals from the question of meaning. A pan-Canadian survey, in early 2017, showed that 19% of respondents did not believe in God and did not adhere to any form of spirituality. David Korzinski, "A spectrum of spirituality: Canadians keep the faith to varying degrees, but few reject it entirely." Angus Reid Institute, http://angusreid.org/religion-in-canada-150/. Retrieved June 13, 2018.

29 Kees Waaijman, *Spirituality: forms, foundations, methods*, vol. 8, Studies in spirituality Supplement (Dudley, Mass: Peeters, 2002), 18–303.

It is hard to imagine "spirituality", which is both the inheritor of traditions and dependent on the answer that must be given, in the singular and as an experience with universal content. Various spiritual traditions respond to a range of calls. As a result, it is possible to propose that the recent biomedical and clinical tradition contextualizes a call heard throughout the modern era, that emphasizes the autonomy of the spiritual subject, individuality, wellbeing and the oceanic feeling, whereas the Christian spiritual traditions respond to a call articulated around the notion of salvation, which can only come from the other.

8.4.2 The axis of alterity

The second axis of the spiritual experience, seen through the prism of radical theology, is articulated around the related characteristics of the uncontainability (section 8.2.1) and excess (section 8.2.3) of an event. As a reminder, uncontainability refers to the fact that the event harboured by a name is not limited by it, while excess is an eruption into daily life and goes beyond the narrow and strict framework of exchange, equivalence and give-and-take. Excess lies in the realm of giving.

While supporting the description of the effects of alterity given by Caputo, I must warn against a possible slippage in the interpretation of excess. In everyday language, the word "excess" is generally associated with a quantitative surplus. This is why it seems important to me to include the vocabulary of excess in the logic of alterity, of otherness, and to talk about the excess of the other, to avoid creating an impression of "more".

Given this fact, alterity leaves traces in many different areas in connection with the spiritual experience.

First, Caputo places alterity at the very heart of the chiasm between insistence and existence, between the call and the response. Tradition is a phenomenon that incorporates a part of otherness, if only because it owes its existence to a call that inhabits it, a call that the response does not exhaust at a particular place and time in history. The call and the event are instances of alterity in the very heart of tradition. The response is something other than the call that triggers it.

Next, Caputo's analysis warns about a danger threatening all traditions and that can be observed regularly: the danger of substituting the response (the tradition) to what triggers and drives it (the call). The problem arises especially when a situated and contextual response is perceived as a universal reality. The most obvious example, in Caputo's opinion, is the metaphysic tradition, inherited from Antiquity, to describe the event that harbours the name (of) "God".

The substitution is also seen in the process used to instrumentalize the call. When the call, which is a promise, becomes a means used in a fight for economic, political or symbolic power, the promissive nature of the event is subverted and subjected.[30] Examples include spiritual discourses that propose submission to an unfair order in return for the promise of eternal happiness in the afterlife. Whether submission is magnified in the context of a social conflict or marital relations (such as submission to a violent spouse), in each case it is a flagrant denial of justice for the victims of a system. If we agree with Caputo's thesis about the chance-based origin of all traditions and all personal vocations—the thesis of their radically historical and circumstantial nature—the substitution I refer to here means "missing the call". Through substitution, the subject or community is placed outside the dynamic that makes a tradition something that is alive.

My third remark concerns the tensions generated within a living tradition by alterity. These tensions are another kind of trace.

The chiasm between the call and the response is a place of tension, and in particular the tension created by the reciprocal irreducibility of the dynamic of effervescence and novelty generated by the call—which embodies the "excessive" nature of the event—and the dynamic of sustainability connected to the institutionalization of a spiritual tradition. The call points to the unknown, to an entry into an unmarked path that is, at the same time, an exit from any logic of reciprocity, equivalence, control or instrumentalization. The call is a place of gratuity and recognition in our personal and collective lives. The event lies outside the realm of things; it resists integration into a political, economic or symbolic "machine". By mentioning the name of Angelus Silesius, a 17th century mystical poet and his aphorism "the rose is without a why",[31] Caputo promotes the idea, iconoclastic for some, that there is no providential order presiding over the destiny of the universe and creation. What lives lives only to live, with no possibility of inscribing a singular life in a universal historic scheme with a defined orientation. Translated into everyday life, this conclusion supports the thesis that the event is something other than institutionalization.

---

30 The question of substitution leads to a reflection on the institutionalization of spiritual life, when considered from the standpoint of theory of the event. What are the conditions for an institutionalization of the spiritual experience that is not purely and simply an instrumentalization to serve power?

31 Silesius Angelus, *Pèlerin chérubinique* = *Cherubinischer Wandersmann* (Aubier: éditions Montaigne, 1946), 107. This echoes the teaching of Meister Eckhart, for whom the universe has no why; cf. Alain de Libera, *Penser au Moyen Âge* (Paris: Seuil, 1991), 346.

8.5 Addressing the articulation between ethics and spirituality

Using the light shed by the idea of the call, I propose a way to address the articulation between ethics and spirituality. The articulation hinges on the hypothesis that both ethics and the spiritual experience are a response to a specific call.

If, as proposed by Ricoeur, ethics is "on the goal of a good life with and for others in just institutions",[32] the insistence contained within it is linked to the experience of good and evil in our individual and collective lives. The call to commitment, responsibility and justice resounds at the core of the ethical life of individuals and communities. It is a call to respond rationally and actively to the question "How can I do good?", which must be asked as soon as a subject is confronted with the tragic dimension of individual and collective life,[33] a dimension that can be deliberately or involuntarily hidden or neglected. The call upsets the banality of everyday life. The tragic dimension of life questions the routines of cultural institutions and the automatisms and reflexes of individual habits. Life, torn between good and evil, and justice and injustice, sets the scene for tragedy where, in many cases, a commitment is made in a complex situation, moral responsibility is needed, and good is aimed for but seldom completely achievable or, *a fortiori*, achieved.

Ethical reflection, like the decisions and actions it gives rise to, is a response to the call that comes from an unknown place, but which resounds where life—in a general sense that includes human life and the cultures where it blossoms— and the conditions that make life possible are made more fragile.

The call to which reflection and spiritual life respond is of another kind. Whether happy or unhappy, the event poses the question of meaning. By creating upheaval, it questions the coherence of individual and collective life. It exceeds expectations; it destabilizes what is agreed and foreseen. The spiritual response to the call of meaning is modulated by the language tradition of the subject. It may occur with the intention of ensuring existential coherence, or under the auspices of grace; the response is deployed gratuitously. The call to gratuitousness is also a call to leave banality behind. It is the insistence of everything that escapes any form of control and any form of subjection. The spiritual calls on us to leave behind the logic of equivalence and the horizon of justice— because of the "logic" of gratuitousness that characterizes giving—and, *a fortiori*,

---

32 Ricoeur, *Soi-même comme un autre*, 202.
33 On the role of tragedy in life and in Christianity, cf. Denis Müller, "Tragique," in *Dictionnaire encyclopédique d'éthique chrétienne*, ed. Laurent Lemoine, Eric Gaziaux, and Denis Müller (Paris: Cerf, 2013): 2004–08.

to leave behind the alienating logic of domination, control, reification and in-strumentalization.

There is therefore a difference between the respective calls of ethics and spi-rituality, and to project spirituality onto ethics can only result from misunder-standing or confusion. If the two calls are different, the logic I have applied up to this point requires that the responses to those calls also be different. This means that the spiritual question must be dealt with separately, without re-ducing it to the sole dimension of self-accomplishment, unlike the main trend in the biomedical and clinical discourse. The spiritual question can be addressed in itself.

I cannot deny that there are some overlapping themes in the field of ethics and spirituality. The question here is to consider this overlapping as a possible configuration for the spirituality-ethics link and not as the only way of viewing it. This is the conclusion I draw from the exploration of the approach of Domi-nique Jacquemin in chapter 6 and of John Caputo in this chapter.

8.6 Spirituality and the event

Addressing the spiritual experience from the standpoint of radical theology pro-duces results that support the reflexive work we have presented so far. However, the outcome for the issues raised by the spiritual experience during illness must be specified. Caputo's reflection focuses on large-scale "objects": the question of the existence of God, the epistemology of the encounter between theology and speculative philosophy,[34] with fundamental physics and the epistemology of sci-ence,[35] etc. His theological project is fundamental in nature. Caputo places his work in the field of theories of theological knowledge, which has an impact on his thinking and on what he thinks about God: "God is not a warranty for a well run world, but the name of a promise, an unkept promise, where every promise is also a risk, a flicker of hope on a suffering planet in a remote corner of the universe. I do not believe in the existence of God but in God's insistence. I do not say God "exists", but that God calls—God calls upon us, like an unwel-come interruption, a quiet but insistent solicitation."[36] This excerpt reveals the fundamental scope of his theological reflection and the resulting relationship with the world.

---

34 Cf. the chapter on continental philosophy and religion in Hegel's work in Caputo, *The Insis-tence of God. A Theology of Perhaps*, 87–116.

35 Caputo, *The Insistence of God. A Theology of Perhaps*, 189–96.

36 Caputo, *The Insistence of God. A Theology of Perhaps*, ix.

Is it possible to transpose, with no further effort, Caputo's epistemological and theoretical framework to objects which, at first sight, appear to be more trivial and routine, such as the biomedical and clinical discourse on spirituality, and even the contextual spiritual experience?

Caputo himself mentions this possibility several times. He recognizes the critical power of the calls heard during the event. For example, the discourses and practices of justice can be deconstructed by emphasizing their irremediably constructed and instituted nature, based on the promise contained within the word "justice". This case, borrowed by Caputo from the work of Derrida,[37] demonstrates one practical and critical aspect of deconstruction.

In his discussion of the displacements that affect the words "grace" and "religion" in the weak theology he proposes, Caputo returns these terms and their respective meanings "to Earth":

> My entire idea is to reclaim religion as an event of this world, to reclaim religion for the world and the world for religion. I have not annulled the religious character of our life but identified its content and extended its reach, by treating it as a name for the event by which life is nourished. In so doing we have redescribed and marked off religion within the boundaries of the world. Religion emerges in response to the promise of the world, to the promise/threat that threads its way through the goods and evils, the joys and sorrows, the loves and enmities of everyday life and knits them together into an inextricable weave [...] This religion without the diversion of otherworldly religion is a religion of a mundane grace, of the grace of this world. A grace is a gift, and life is a gift of time and death, the grace of an instant, a mortal grace, not an otherworldly one, a grace that finds words in a weak theology of the world.[38]

Whether or not one agrees with the resolutely immanentist nature of Caputo's approach to religion[39] and grace, it opens the way for further research where the "tools" can be applied to the "objects" of the spiritual traditions. The conceptual framework proposed by Caputo leaves nothing outside the reach of analysis and critical thought. Each of the fundamental dimensions of human life in turn enters the laboratory of deconstructive analysis: "natality, mortality, carnality, terrestriality, materiality—hitherto 'ultimates', the outer limits, unquestioned necessary horizons of thinking—come into question as contingent limits, sur-

---

37 Caputo, *The Weakness of God. A Theology of the Event*, 27–28.
38 Caputo, *The Insistence of God. A Theology of Perhaps*, 247.
39 Caputo uses the word "religion" in the singular. In my view there is a discrepancy between his use of religion in the singular and his theory that refutes the universality of concepts and meanings.

passable horizons, inscribed within the horizon without horizon of 'perhaps'."[40] In short, under the rule of "perhaps", very little is left unquestioned.

In short, if life and its precariousness, along with religion and grace, can be analyzed and discussed under the light shed by deconstruction, the same holds true for the spiritual experience during illness. In addition, this specific spiritual experience is located at the meeting-point of life, religion and grace, as understood by Caputo, which corresponds to what I have called here the lay-humanist tradition of spirituality, just as is it located at the meeting-point of religion and grace as understood by the Christian spiritual traditions. I must also add the fact that the spiritual experience during illness is a subject of constant institutionalized concern in the healthcare world, as described in the first part of this book, which highlights the constructed nature of the spiritual experience and its integration into the healthcare world. We must also not forget that healthcare institutions have become a major component of social life with clear normative power over our lives, in the sense that they have the power to determine the direction of thoughts and actions—in short, they help define what is an ideal life, good life or valuable life.[41] This consecrated status in the contemporary mindset supports the choice of Caputo's theoretical framework for use in analyzing the spiritual experience during illness.

8.7 Conclusion to chapter eight

This chapter had a modest objective. The goal was to draw inspiration from the radical theology of John Caputo to verify the potential of his work to stimulate a theological reflection on the spiritual experience that challenged the *a priori* of the biomedical and clinical tradition and the theological interpretations that support it. I should point out that the exercise involved rebutting the reductive discourse that makes the spiritual experience an object of care or a care adjuvant. For this purpose, the reflexive approach I propose has to call into question the most fundamental theoretical presuppositions. A superficial analysis would not be sufficient—I had to go as far as the presuppositions on the "nature" of the spiritual experience. This is the level at which the references to the work of Caputo are relevant. By presenting a fundamental theological reflection that is completely different from the metaphysical gesture inherited from Antiquity, Ca-

---

40 Caputo, *The Insistence of God. A Theology of Perhaps*, 259.
41 I should repeat here the common observation that good health, and practices to maintain or regain good health, have equivalent status to salvation and the salvational practices promoted by religious groups.

puto offers a conceptual system that can generate another comprehension of spiritual life, able to change the generally-held point of view on the spiritual experience during illness and way in which it is taken into account in healthcare.

What emerges from the discussion in this chapter is that the spiritual experience during illness is far more diversified than admitted in the biomedical and clinical literature. Some of the theological intuitions developed in Caputo's work can be used to consider the spiritual experience as a highly complex, highly volatile, multi-faceted reality that hides many surprises, and can even call into question various presuppositions held in its respect in the healthcare world. This will form the subject-matter of the next chapter.

9 Spiritual life and traditions during illness

It is now time to complete the reflection presented in the second part of this book, by looking again at the expression of spiritual life during illness using the interpretive keys provided by Caputo.

9.1 Illness and the event

It is easy to see that several of the descriptive categories of an event defined by Caputo are applicable to illness. Stating that illness is partly event-based does not mean that it is providential in the sense that it is intended by Providence, the Supreme Being or the organizing principle of the universe. Like an event, illness is not an element in a grander scheme. Even though, in a table of clinical diseases, an illness may appear to belong to a certain order—for example, the symptoms of typhus are not similar to those of Creutzfeldt-Jakob disease—this does not mean that, phenomenologically speaking, each illness is part of an order that is larger, that gives it meaning, or that endows it with a share of intelligibility and rationality. In short, the internal coherence of a table of diseases does not guarantee that it becomes part of the universe of meaning. Illness is anything but an order. After this reminder, I intend to address the event-based aspect of illness by discussing its relationship to meaning and time, and as a call.

9.1.1 Meaning

Illness is an irruption; it ruptures banality or the normal order. This is how it is experienced by people whose health is threatened. If this were not so, the sick would not be complaining "Why? Why me? What have I done to deserve this?"

From the point of view of meaning, illness is characterized by a basic ambiguity that opens the door to interpretation. The fact that illness has no meaning does not prevent the sick from legitimately seeking to give it one. In the absence of a predetermined meaning, illness is open to the interpretation of the person who is experiencing it. Although illness may be seen negatively by this person, and by the people around him or her, sometimes it will be given a positive attribute, for example when it is seen as a key moment when choices must be made that are then interpreted as being liberating and beneficial. Similarly, illness may

https://doi.org/10.1515/9783110638950-010

provide an opportunity to develop unsuspected personal potential, without this being considered as resignation or rationalization.

The range of subjective interpretations of illness should be compared to what Caputo has to say about the event as a promise and as a "reality" that can bring evil: "The excess of the event is not necessarily good news. Evil, which I will describe as irreparably reserved time, without the possibility of compensation, also exhibits this excess. [...] Accordingly, an event can result in a disintegrating destablilization and a diminished recontextualization just as well as it can create an opening of the future."[1]

9.1.2 Time

The irruption of illness into a person's life takes place in the *kairos*. It creates a tear in the fabric of a human life. The life story—both temporal and narrative—is marked and divided into before- and after-illness segments. The normal and ongoing course of life is interrupted. However, nothing prevents a restructuring of the life story around the illness in order to restore a level of "normality" and even "banality" during the morbid event, whether of short, medium or long duration. For example, a long period of stability with respect to the symptoms can be experienced as *chronos*,[2] ordinary time with no upsets except those caused by the illness.

9.1.3 The call

Last, illness can be considered as the vector for a call. As we will see later, the call arising from an episode of illness is both ethical and spiritual, although the two aspects remain separate. Care is a response to the call embodied in the illness. As a result, it is possible to understand the illness/care binomial as a concrete example of the event/response pair theorized by Caputo.

In short, the event and the illness share some facets that reveal a structural homology, in other words a similar form, at least in part. Illness is a quasi-event because of its excess, its basically indeterminate meaning, the temporal and narrative effects it induces and the correlation of the illness/care binomial with the event/response binomial.

---

1 Caputo, *The Weakness of God. A Theology of the Event*, 5.
2 See section 8.2.5 of chapter 8.

The fact that the illness is a quasi-event encourages me to pursue in the same vein to analyze the spiritual experience during illness. For this, I will consider the biomedical and clinical spiritual tradition, as well as the Christian spiritual traditions, in light of the insistence/existence, call/response chiasm proposed by Caputo.

9.2 The spiritual traditions and responses to the call

The status of illness as a quasi-event opens up the possibility of considering all the spiritual traditions (religious, biomedical and clinical, lay, etc.) present in a healthcare institution as responses to that which makes itself heard during the illness event. The call is the call of personal vulnerability, the fragility of life, and the precarious balance between an individual and his or her environment, all characteristics induced by the quasi-event of illness. The call is also a call with an ethical dimension in terms of solidarity with the sick person, a call to clearly reaffirm the person's humanity despite the illness and the damage it inflicts, a call to be responsible for someone who is vulnerable and fragile.[3]

Two responses to this call can be heard. The first is ethico-moral in nature. It was formerly embodied in the Hippocratic Oath and then, from the 1960s, in the institutionalization of bioethics, more specifically in clinical ethics. What is the best way to dispense care? This is the central question in clinical ethics, and is also found at the heart of organizational ethics in healthcare institutions, in particular in the form of institutional codes of conduct that set out the rights and duties of patients and care providers in the care relationship[4] or, in other cases, the rights, duties and responsibilities of the institution itself. The bioethical reflection is therefore part of a long tradition of ethico-moral thought and action triggered by the quasi-event of illness.

However, this is not the only form of response to the appeal that comes from the quasi-event of illness. The spiritual discourses used in Western healthcare institutions are also a clear response to illness. They reflect a range of world views and propose concrete actions to social actors—including patients—in the healthcare institutions, whether lay or religious, to provide a framework for illness, dying and death. Traditionally, these responses were provided by religious institutions in the form of rites, theological explanations of the role and meaning of

---

3 Paul Ricoeur, "Le concept de responsabilité. Essai d'analyse sémantique," in *Le juste I* (Paris: Éditions Esprit, 1995): 69.
4 Codes of professional conduct and charters of patients' rights, where these forms of regulation exist, should also be added.

illness, religious forms of consolation, etc., but they now come from other social authorities, and in particular the healthcare institutions themselves.

The "responsorial" status of the spiritual traditions identified by theology of the event is not the only benefit derived from this explanation. The analysis framework inspired by the work of Caputo can also be used to confirm the anthropological point of view discussed in chapter 7. The application of the theology of the event confirms the fundamental historicity of the spiritual traditions in the healthcare world. The wide range of religious spiritual traditions that deal with the meaning of illness and death, along with the variety of pastoral practices applied, bear witness to a constant feature of the history of spiritual practices and discourses in the West, namely the taking into account of the socio-cultural context by the various groups producing spiritual discourses. It goes without saying that the biomedical and clinical spiritual tradition is also a historically and culturally situated tradition, as discussed earlier. The theology of the event is not limited to an identification of the historical nature of the spiritual traditions, since it also emphasizes that they are a response to a call or, at least, to the insistent features of the quasi-event of illness. The spiritual call comes from illness and death, both in the lives of individuals and in the life of society. This is why, in my opinion, it is important to distinguish between the call for responsibility, which generates an ethico-moral response, and the call for meaning, which generates a spiritual response.

The irruption of illness triggers a crisis of meaning that generally leads to a "loss of general reference frameworks and loss of control over one's own life."[5] This, in turn, leads to the questions "Why?" and "What for?", respectively concerning the cause and the meaning of the illness, asked by the sick person and his or her relatives. The crisis of meaning is based on the fact that the illness itself is nonsensical, in other words that it has no meaning in itself, even if the episode of morbidity is part of a causal chain. Whatever the cause of a cancer (smoking or involuntary exposure to cancerous products, etc.), it has no meaning in itself. Because of its absurd nature, illness raises the question of meaning and leads to an attempt by the person concerned to place it against a horizon of meaning of some kind. From a narrative point of view, assigning a meaning to the episode of morbidity involves reconciling the discordance of illness with the concordance of the story, in this case the patient's life story.[6] In this way,

---

5 Lazare Benaroyo, "Éthique et herméneutique du soin," in *La philosophie du soin Éthique, médecine et société*, ed. Lazare Benaroyo et al. (Paris: Presses universitaires de France, 2010): 26.
6 Jobin, *Des religions à la spiritualité. Une appropriation biomédicale du religieux dans l'hôpital*, 92–94; Guy Jobin, "Quand narrer, c'est (re)construire: intrigue et récit en temps de maladie," in *L'intrigue dans le récit biblique*, ed. Anne Pasquier, Daniel Marguerat, and André Wénin, Biblio-

the illness is connected to other previous situations which, in a way, give it a framework. It can then be inserted into the weave of the biographical journey, which already contains sedimentary meanings that can be reactivated. This, of course, depends on the effort made by the sick person and his or her close circle. There is no guarantee or requirement that a meaning will be found for the episode of morbidity.

However, it is possible that the event will cause so much disturbance that it leads to a restructuring of some or all of the patient's system of meaning. The 1991 film "The Doctor", starring William Hurt, depicts this kind of shift in the perspective of a cancer-stricken physician. So, the role played by the spiritual traditions will be to support the search for meaning undertaken by the patient or his or her close circle, or even by caregivers.[7] The patient can use his or her traditions to confer meaning on the episode, or may begin a search for a meaning that appears more relevant than those immediately available.

9.3 Spiritual traditions in the healthcare world

The event-like nature of illness is revealed thanks to use of the theoretical framework based on theology of the event. We can now use the same approach to examine the two main families of spiritual discourse present in the healthcare world: biomedical and clinical discourses, and religious discourses.

Probably the only consensus among researchers working on spirituality in healthcare concerns the impossibility of identifying and obtaining a consensus position on a definition of spirituality. This is also my observation. However, the generally recognized impossibility of achieving a consensus definition does not mean that the existing definitions are divergent, or that each is specific to a given situation. Despite their diversity they are not irreducible. I suggest that they can be grouped into two major families. The first is made up of definitions in which spirituality is conceived of as an inner-worldly phenomenon, intrinsic to human nature, and is therefore seen to be strictly human with its source in human nature. The second is made up to definitions in which spirituality is seen as a manifestation of alterity in human nature, whether the "other" is

---

theca Ephemeridum Theologicarum Lovaniensis, 237 (Leuven: Peeters, 2010): 87–107; Paul Ricoeur, *Temps et récit. T.2 La configuration dans le récit de fiction*, Points Essais, 228 (Paris: Seuil, 1984), 41.

7 In the latter case, this occurs when a caregiver proposes a spiritual or religious interpretation of a medical incident, for example by suggesting to the parents of a still-born child that they are now under the care of an angel.

seen as a form of transcendence (as it is in monotheist and polytheist religions) or as an intra-worldly force that is greater than any individual (Nature, the Cosmos, etc.). It appears clear to me that most of the biomedical and clinical discourses about spirituality belong to the first group, while the religious discourses belong to the second group.

9.3.1 Biomedical and clinical discourses[8]

Based on the theoretical framework used in this chapter, two key facts emerge from the analysis of the biomedical discourses on spirituality.

9.3.1.1 Wellbeing as a call requiring a spiritual response

My analysis of the biomedical discourses on spirituality shows the structuring strength of the wellbeing category in the clinical approach to spirituality. There can be no doubt that the biomedical culture shares the notion of wellbeing with Western spiritual culture. But, as I attempted to explain in the first part of this book, wellbeing has acquired a central theoretical status and a crucial operationality in biomedical thought and clinical practice. Given these special circumstances, the biomedical spiritual discourse may be considered as a response to a call, the call for wellbeing, that has all the appearances of a fundamental meaning which, once institutionalized, provides precise directions and rules for living. Although crucial, this finding is not enough. We must look in more depth at the question by identifying the presuppositions that guide this conception of spirituality.

9.3.1.2 Presuppositions

By highlighting, once again, the constructed nature of every spiritual response and its undeniable anthropological dimension, the theology of the event asks us to identify the presuppositions that structure the biomedical interpretation of the spiritual experience during illness. Two presuppositions emerge clearly from an analytical standpoint.

The first is the ontological nature of the relationship between salvation and health, which I have already discussed in the chapter 3. In the biomedical approach, and for many Westerners, health is the current figure of salvation, in

---

8 To streamline the text in this section I have shortened this label to "biomedical discourses".

other words a representation of the ideal state to which human beings (should) aspire. The power and attraction of this belief is such that it underlies the search for human longevity and the utopia of a transhumanist triumph over death, for example. Without going as far as the transhumanists, the biomedical spiritual discourse still relies on identifying an inner-worldly form of salvation in the idea of good spiritual health.

The second clear presupposition is reflected in the pragmatism displayed in the biomedical discourse. By pragmatism, I mean the conception of spirituality based on its effects on the patient, on the care relationship and on the healthcare institution. In addition to the fact that spirituality is an "object" in health policies[9] and an "object" of research in the biomedical sciences, it is also the vector for one of the major concerns for healthcare institutions: humanization.[10] To recapitulate, there are three themes in the discourse about humanization in the healthcare world. Moving from the particular to the general, the first theme concerns the care relationship. Here, humanization results from the clinical focus on the repercussions of illness in all dimensions of human life. In other words, the holistic delivery of care (whether multi- or interdisciplinary) is both a vector and a sign of the humanization of care.[11] The next two themes concern the humanization of organizations. First, a correlation has been established between job satisfaction and spirituality in the workplace. One research project reports that "the research results indicate that there is a positive relationship between workplace spirituality and job satisfaction. These findings deepen the understanding of personal spirituality, organizational spirituality, and job satisfaction. They bring new insights into the significant role which spirituality plays in the context of the workplace."[12] Next, organizational research has shown "a sense of community and meaningful work are the most important dimensions of workplace spirituality in health care."[13]

These few examples show that the spirituality mobilized by the biomedical and clinical discourse is perceived as a force where efforts to transform practice

---

9 WHO, *La Charte de Bangkok pour la promotion de la santé à l'heure de la mondialisation*.
10 This was mentioned briefly in chapter 6, section 6.7.1.
11 Bjarnason, "Nursing, religiosity, and end-of-life care: interconnections and implications"; Ronald A. Carson, "Engaged humanities: moral work in the precincts of medicine," *Perspect Biol Med* 50, no. 3 (2007); Sasser and Puchalski, "The humanistic clinician: traversing the science and art of health care"; Isaiah D. Wexler and Benjamin W. Corn, "An existential approach to oncology: meeting the needs of our patients," *Current Opinion in Supportive & Palliative Care* 6, no. 2 (2012).
12 van der Walt and de Klerk, "Workplace spirituality and job satisfaction".
13 Heidi Pirkola, Piia Rantakokko, and Marjo Suhonen, "Workplace spirituality in health care: an integrated review of the literature," *J Nurs Manag* 24, no. 7 (2016).

and institutional functions can obtain support. Since spirituality is considered to be something of substance, in other words as a dimension able to be modified by a clinical intervention or mobilized as part of a therapy, it takes only one more step to make it a potential force for change.

The pragmatic nature of the biomedical spiritual discourse is immediately identifiable when it is compared to the gratuitousness of the event and the call it engenders.[14] The gratuitousness or gift of the event highlights the gap between the call and the response in terms of humanization. There is undeniable tension between the alterity-excess-uncontainability triad of the call and the response in terms of humanization, which presupposes aims, goals and strategies designed to modify individual and collective behaviour.

I can only repeat that it is commendable to want to transform and improve the operation of healthcare institutions with the aim of improving the wellbeing of patients and workers. This is not the problem. Instead, the problem is created by the need to rely on spirituality in an organizational transformation project or strategy for change. The "spirituality and humanization of care organization" casefile shows the importance placed by institutions on the effects of spiritual life and its institutionalization. The spirituality and care relations "casefile" shows that, once again, the effect on individuals and on quality of care is a key argument used to justify and legitimate the role of spirituality in the clinical world. In short, whether spirituality is seen as one factor among many in achieving care goals, or as one factor among many in transforming healthcare organizations, the same pragmatic "spirit" is involved.

To conclude, a juxtaposition of the theology of the event and the biomedical spiritual discourse shows that the discourse is, like any spiritual language tradition, a response to a call. It is a genuine tradition. The theology of the event also makes it possible to identify the fundamental aim of the biomedical response to the call for wellbeing.

9.3.2 Traditional discourses

The traditional spiritual discourses are just as open to analysis using the theology of the event. The fact that these discourses are connected to a specific religious tradition does not make them immune from critical scrutiny. It is by virtue of their status as a response to a call that analysis is "applicable" to their case. Four main remarks can be made.

---

14 Cf. chapter 8, section 8.4.2.

9.3.2.1 The call of salvation, in the form of an analogy

The question of salvation is, here too, of primary importance. However, the main difference between the Christian spiritual response and the biomedical and clinical spiritual response is that, traditionally, health is not seen as salvation *in itself*, but as an *analogy* of salvation. A glance at some of the founding texts of Christianity makes this clear. In the Gospels, a return to health is an approximate image of divine pardon for sins and of the gracious restoration it effects in each person who receives it. Health is a striking and even eloquent image, but it remains an image, an incomplete representation of what grace, God's gift, can achieve. This difference between the religious discourse, which sees health as an image of salvation, and the biomedical discourse, which sees health and salvation as being equivalent, is fundamental. And I believe that because of this difference it is plausible to divide the spiritual discourses into two main families, as mentioned above.

To the relationship between salvation and health must be added the question of temporality.[15] The timeline along which Christian spiritual life is deployed includes a period beyond human time, whether *chronos* or *kairos*. A classic example of this is the spiritual experience of a patient who relies on a belief in life after death in deciding whether to refuse or cease treatment. This has been observed in the dialysis sector for people with end stage renal disease.[16] When a patient's spiritual life and beliefs encourage him or her to consider ceasing treatment, it seems reasonable to believe that the decision is influenced by the fact that the patient has a representation of some sort of survival in the afterlife. In this case, caregivers suggesting persevering with the treatment, based on a timeline that is limited to the time available to provide care, may be dismayed. In this example, the patient and the caregivers find themselves at odds with respect to the scope of the decision that must be made.

9.3.2.2 Diversity of experiences and traditions

Theology of the event makes it possible to recognize the diversity of spiritual experiences in Christianity. The fact that diversity exists is evident when one looks

---

15 This question was discussed in chapter 5, section 5.1.2.3.

16 Davison and Jhangri, "Existential and religious dimensions of spirituality and their relationship with health-related quality of life in chronic kidney disease"; Kimmel et al., "ESRD patient quality of life: symptoms, spiritual beliefs, psychosocial factors, and ethnicity"; Patel et al., "Psychosocial variables, quality of life, and religious beliefs in ESRD patients treated with hemodialysis"; Spinale et al., "Spirituality, social support, and survival in hemodialysis patients"; Tanyi and Werner, "Adjustment, spirituality, and health in women on hemodialysis".

at the contingencies of time and place, in short the circumstances, in which new spiritual movements emerge and grow. Christianity includes a range of spiritual experiences, and is found in a range of cultures where the message of salvation proposed by the Gospels has taken hold. It is important to note that this diversity is also visible in each new generation of believers, when various forms of spiritual life are found alongside each other. The call leads, perhaps inevitably, to a range of responses over the course of history, but also in specific periods.

9.3.2.3 The diversity of institutional forms
Given the diversity of experiences and contexts, the diversity of institutional forms comes as no surprise. A spiritual experience can become institutionalized as a school of spirituality[17] (such as the Jesuit tradition of discernment of spirits), as a counter-cultural spirituality (such as spiritualities of liberation) or as a quasi-professional form of spiritual accompaniment (like *Spiritual Care* in North America and in English-speaking countries), and all these forms illustrate the inherent diversity of responses to the call.

The diversity of institutional traditions and forms reflects another important aspect of the theology of the event, which is the incontainability of an event by its name. The event is always other (this is how I interpret the excess discussed by Caputo); it cannot be reduced to the language-based and institutional mechanisms used to give it concrete expression at a particular point in human history. Any sedimentation of the event in a specific tradition will inevitably be partial. In other words, there will never be, by definition, mechanisms that are better than others. There are only, *prima faciae*, the various responses to the call. Nevertheless, the call is there, tirelessly.

9.3.2.4 A question of recognition
The diversity of the responses to the call emphasizes the inevitable alterity that inhabits pluralistic societies. Wherever we look, we are always facing the other. Theology of the event takes into account the moral and religious plurality of Western societies and reflects, generally and about itself, about ways to integrate plurality in the vision of the world it proposes.

One of the concrete and immediate effects of this openness to alterity displayed by theology of the event is recognition for the loss of the monopoly of religious discourses over the spiritual experience, and recognition of the existence

---

17 Waaijman, *Spirituality: forms, foundations, methods*, 8.

of the main families of spiritual discourses. The religious traditions that left their mark on Western culture are no longer the only ones to "address spirituality". However, recognition of plurality does not prevent analysis and criticism of those traditions, or discussions between spiritual traditions. On the contrary, it reflects the contemporary quest for truth.[18]

In concrete terms, this means that the biomedical and clinical conception of the spiritual experience during illness is neither more nor less legitimate than any other conception. It offers a view of the patient experience that is not rooted in the same material as the spiritual traditions that stem from Christianity. Like them, however, it must look critically at its own sources, at the institutional mechanisms that update it, and at the strengths and weaknesses that run through it. The biomedical and clinical spiritual discourse is a reality that, because of its normative strength, must be examine from a critical standpoint, like any form of institutionalized standard.

9.4 Consequences for clinical practice

I would like to end this chapter with a discussion of some of the potential impacts of the preceding points on clinical practice and on the training of biomedical and clinical practitioners.

9.4.1 Professional caregivers

My first remark concerns the attention given by caregivers to the diversity of their patients' spiritual experiences. The interweaving of various traditions of spiritual language and practices, together with the primacy of individuals and their freedom of belief as guaranteed in law-based societies, puts paid to the idea of a single, universal and canonic form of spiritual experience during illness. Life, in general, and spiritual life, in particular, can take so many different forms during a human lifetime that it is unrealistic to try to enclose them in models that are unresponsive to diversity.

The corollary of this recommendation regarding clinical practice concerns the training given to caregivers. The younger generation is already less familiar than the baby-boomer generation with religious and spiritual matters, and this experiential trend is accelerating in secularized societies. As we saw above,

---

18 John D. Caputo, *Truth* (New York: Penguin Books, 2013).

the group of people who are "without religion and without spirituality" is growing at a faster pace than those who are "spiritual but not religious" or "religious". The mixing of the population thanks to immigration, which increases the religious and cultural diversification of the host society and multiplies the number of patients' religious and spiritual profiles, must also be taken into account. One of the challenges involved is how to train new generations of caregivers about the meaning of the religious or spiritual experience in individual or collective lives. Obviously, training is not an opportunity for conversion. It has a professional goal: to ensure that care providers can respond suitably to the "instruction" to take patients' spiritual or religious experience into account—an instruction that is increasingly heard—regardless of their own personal views on the matter. This is the key issue. They must be motivated by no beliefs other than those that guide their professional actions.

The second recommendation also concerns a gap, this time the gap caused by tension between the world vision guiding a patient's spiritual experiences, on the one hand, and the biomedical and clinical discourse, on the other. The issue is not the gap itself, but the judgment made about that gap, given the normative weight attributed to the biomedical and clinical discourse. Here, there is a double risk: either to "discount" the patient's spiritual experience when it differs from the clinical conception, or to impose a foreign belief on the patient under the cover of a professional or expert opinion. The training given to care providers must allow them to establish a critical distance with the normative nature of the biomedical and clinical discourse and with their own beliefs. There is nothing alarming in this, since it is already a requisit of professional conduct.

9.4.2 Researchers

Research, too, introduces normativity that shapes the discourses on the spiritual experience during illness. As in any field of knowledge, research formats the object of its scrutiny.[19]

How, or in what way, are researchers sensitive to the methodological biases that can mask the multitude of patients' spiritual experiences? This is the question. It is not connected to the improvement of care, which I identified above as the pragmatic side of this research field.

---

19 Bruno Latour, *Pandora's Hope. Essays on the Reality of Science Studies* (Cambridge Ma.: Harvard University Press, 1999).

The question is a reflexive one about the way in which the clinical research world constructs the objet it examines and about the proposals for the concrete mobilization of the object in clinical practice. To maintain the reflection requires the development of a research field to elucidate the mechanisms used to produce knowledge about spirituality during illness. The approach must be deployed differently from the pragmatic approach mainly used in the field.

9.4.3 Chaplains

In addition to providing spiritual accompaniment for patients, families and care providers who request it, chaplains have a role in providing ongoing training. Who is in a better position than a chaplain to present and remind people of the diversity of the spiritual experience during illness? Who is in a better position to convey, or even translate, the patients' spiritual experiences in a language that will allow care providers to understand the content of the spiritual experiences they can support with their clinical skills?

As we can see, the new awareness of the diversity of spiritual experiences during illness and the impossibility of reducing them to a single biomedical and clinical model leaves room for chaplains, beyond their primary work of accompanying relatives and families. Their work also includes giving training to care providers about the issues of spiritual and religious diversity.

9.5 Conclusion to chapter nine

By looking anew at the elements of the spirituality/health question using the framework for analysis provided by theology of the event, we can both reiterate and extend the conclusions of chapter 7 on spiritual anthropology, by highlighting the impossibility of reducing the spiritual experience to the single conception promoted by the biomedical and clinical world. Language and traditions of language have a matricial status with respect to experience—they guide ways of thinking, speaking of and addressing the spiritual terms in practical terms. It could even be said that without language and the traditions of language, there can be no response to the call.

In light of current trends in the biomedical literature on spirituality in the clinical world, it is important to offer criticism that avoids undue praise, but is not pointlessly sterile. The reality is that the biomedical world has a strong hold, and will not let go simply because it is criticized, whatever the anchor point for the criticism: sociological, anthropological, or theological. This statement does not mean that all criticism is in vain.

The critique I propose in this book is designed to show that the biomedical language is a tradition of language, sharing the strengths and weaknesses of its time, like any other tradition of language and, *a fortiori*, the traditions of spiritual language.

Now that we have reached the end of this chapter, readers may wonder if the journey was worth the effort. Have we merely shifted the search for a universal foundation of spiritual life from an experiential foundation to a language-based foundation? Is the task, now, to identify a universal language of spiritual life that can smooth out the differences between the lay and denominational forms of language used to describe spirituality? These reactions would fail to take into account the structuring nature of language in understanding spiritual life and its manifestations. The action of looking for the foundation of spirituality is itself dependent on a tradition of language, whether we like it or not.

In short, considering the nature of illness as a quasi-event, in light of Caputo's work, makes it possible to focus on the crucial anthropological and theological issues that run through and structure the practices and discourses used to take the spiritual life into account in the clinical world. In fact, the comparison of the theology of the event with current spiritual accompaniment practices in the healthcare community is not intended to determine what spirituality is, but rather to hear the call harboured within its name.

10 Conclusion

The biomedical and clinical focus on the spiritual experience during illness, al-though relatively recent, still has all the characteristics of a process that is as old as human society itself: the process of institutionalization. The practices, dis-courses, norms, and representations generated by a conscious and deliberate ef-fort to take spirituality into account in clinical practice are, in fact, visible traces of the constant quest to humanize healthcare institutions.

However, this effort to integrate the spiritual experience, and the "mecha-nisms" put in place to achieve that goal, may fail to fully achieve the underlying regulatory intent of all institutionalization processes. It might encounter resis-tance.

As shown here, this "resistance" is inherent in the "object" itself. Spiritual life is hard to institutionalize. This observation is confirmed, eloquently and clearly, by two thousand years of Christianity and the profusion of diverse spiri-tual propositions it has generated. In fact, it would be better to state that spiri-tual life continually overflows the frameworks created to confine it within an in-stitutional environment, of whatever kind. Without being the polar opposite of institutional life, spiritual life contains a share of unavailability, in other words it cannot submit entirely to regulation by an institution. From this point of view, spirituality is the institution's "other", the face of alterity in a human organization.

As I emphasized several times in this book, the "otherness" of spiritual life depends on the tradition of language to make itself heard and appreciated. Spi-ritual alterity, as expressed through language, is also a condition on which spi-ritual life can be welcomed into the healthcare world. It is in and through lan-guage—in the broad meaning of a relationship to the world that includes mindsets, speech, gestures and action—that the spiritual experience can be seen and understood. It is tempting to paraphrase the old adage, and to state that "outside language, there is no contact with spiritual experience!"

We have seen that there are many different traditions of language in the healthcare world, even though, as I have suggested, they can be divided into two main groups: the humanist language traditions, and the traditions that in-clude a form of transcendence. We have also seen that the biomedical and clin-ical world conceives of spiritual life separately from its underlying language-based nature. It is thought of, and addressed directly, as an experience of imme-diacy (the oceanic feeling described by Liogier), an experience of a direct con-nection between the person and a spiritual source, whether oneself, God, Nature, etc. This is one of the paradoxes of contemporary "spiritual culture": ignoring

https://doi.org/10.1515/9783110638950-011

the language-based, traditional, social, and in short institutionalized, nature of spiritual life just as it is being integrated into lay institutions that also, I should point, play a central role in social life.

The Western healthcare institutions participate in the spiritual movement that structures our shared culture, while adding their own particularities to the shared conception of spirituality: medicalization, pragmatism, measurement of the effects of spiritual life, etc. We have seen, throughout this book, the influence that the normativity of the healthcare world has on the representations, practices and discourses connected to spiritual life.

The promises and limits embodied in this new openness have been examined from various standpoints, including that of theological reflection, of course, but also from an anthropological and sociological point of view. Like any social phenomenon, the reception of spiritual life by the clinical world is complex, and must be examined from all possible angles in order to gain an accurate understanding.

In my view it was necessary to criticize, in as nuanced a way as possible, the goals and the methods used by stakeholders in the healthcare world to understand spiritual life during illness and apply it for care purposes. I believe it is important to describe the context for the emergence of health-based discourses and practices about spiritual life, to identify what I consider to be their main driving forces and, above all, to endeavour to show that this is not the only possible discourse, even if it is the most commonly stated and most widely heard. The thesis I have defended here is that spiritual life can only be understood to its full extent if it is addressed as what it is: a language-based phenomenon, in the strict hermeneutic meaning of the term. The corollary of this thesis is that the spiritual experience is expressed and understood within a tradition of language, and depends on that tradition. In the current state of Western societies, where secularism and religious plurality predominate, spiritual life makes itself manifest in many different ways that cannot be reduced to a lower common denominator.

Some readers may think that the critical examination presented here is driven by nostalgia for a time when the religious traditions were the sole bearers of the codes and keys needed to interpret spiritual life. In fact, I am not proposing that we return to the time when religious tradition was the dominant force in healthcare institutions or when, since we are dealing with nostalgia, medicine relied on wooden stethoscopes. My goal was to establish a critical distance with the biomedical and clinical discourse on spiritual life during illness solely in order to highlight the diversity of ways in which spiritual life is expressed. This diversity must be understood as an effect of the anthropological anchoring that makes language the medium through which spiritual life is expressed.

Credits

I thank the following publications for granting permission to reproduce excerpts from previously published material:

Underwood, Lynn G. & Teresi, Jeanne A. "The Daily Spiritual Experience Scale: Development, theoretical description, reliability, exploratory factor analysis, and preliminary construct validity using health related data." *Annals of Behavioral Medicine*, 24, no. 1 (Winter 2002): 26, reproduced at p. 59 – 60.

Éditions Jésuites for the excerpt from Monod-Zorzi, Stéfanie. *Soins aux personnes âgées. Intégrer la spiritualité?*, Soins et spiritualités. Edited by Eckhard Frick and Cosette Odier. Vol. 2, Bruxelles: Lumen vitae, 2012: 55, reproduced at p. 61 – 62.

Éditions Elsevier Masson for the excerpt from NANDA International. "Détresse spirituelle." In *Diagnostics infirmiers. Définitions et classification 2012 – 2014*, Issy-les-Moulineaux, 2013: 439, reproduced at p. 49 – 50.

American Family Physician for the excerpt from Anandarajah, Gowri and Ellen Hight, "Spirituality and medical practice: using the HOPE questions as a practical tool for spiritual assessment", *American Family Physician* 63, no. 1 (Jan 01 2001): 87, reproduced at p. 55 – 56.

Acknowledgments

I thank the donators and the Board of Directors of the Religion, spirituality and Health Research Chair, for the funding necessary to realise this publication.

https://doi.org/10.1515/9783110638950-012

Bibliography

Adler, Rolf H. "Engel's biopsychosocial model is still relevant today." *Journal of Psychosomatic Research* 67, no. 6 (Dec 2009): 607–11.

Al-Arabi, Safaa. "Quality of Life : Subjective." *Nephrology Nursing Journal : Journal of the American Nephrology Nurses' Association* 33, no. 3 (2006): 285–94.

Allard, Maxime. "De la possibilité d'entendre du 'spirituel' en fin de vie." In *Spiritualités et biomédecine Enjeux d'une intégration*, edited by Guy Jobin, Jean-Marc Charron and Michel Nyabenda, 3–20. Québec: Presses de l'Université Laval, 2013.

Alvarez, Ana S., Marco Pagani, and Paolo Meucci. "The clinical application of the biopsychosocial model in mental health: a research critique." *American journal of physical medicine & rehabilitation* 91, no. 13 Suppl 1 (Feb 2012): S173–80.

Ambroselli, Claire, Anne Fagot-Largeault, and Christiane Sinding. "Avant-propos." In *La fabrique du corps humain*, 9–16. Arles: Actes sud/INSERM, 1987.

Anandarajah, Gowri, and Ellen Hight. "Spirituality and medical practice: using the HOPE questions as a practical tool for spiritual assessment." *American Family Physician* 63, no. 1 (Jan 01 2001): 81–9.

Angelus, Silesius. *Pèlerin chérubinique = Cherubinischer Wandersmann.* Aubier: éditions Montaigne, 1946.

Appleby, Brenda Margaret, and Nuala P. Kenny. "Relational personhood, social justice and the common good: Catholic contributions toward a public health ethics." *Christian Bioethics* 16, no. 3 (2010): 296–313.

Ariès, Philippe. *L'homme devant la mort 2. La mort ensauvagée.* Points Histoire 83. Paris: Seuil, 1977.

Aristote. *Éthique de Nicomaque.* Translated by Jean Voilquin. Paris: Gallimard Flammarion, 1992.

Dictionnaire de spiritualité ascétique et mystique. Paris: Beauchesne, 1935.

Astrow, Alan B., Christina M. Puchalski, and Daniel P. Sulmasy. "Religion, spirituality, and health care: social, ethical, and practical considerations." *Am J Med* 110, no. 4 (Mar 2001): 283–7.

Asurmendy, Jesus. "Sagesse." In *Dictionnaire encyclopédique d'éthique chrétienne*, edited by Laurent Lemoine, Eric Gaziaux and Denis Müller. Paris: Cerf, 2013.

Baertschi, Bernard. "Valeurs et vertus." In *Introduction à l'éthique Penser, croire, agir*, edited by Jean-Daniel Causse and Denis Müller, 177–97. Genève: Labor et Fides, 2009.

Baldacchino, Donia R. "Nursing competencies for spiritual care." *Journal of Clinical Nursing* 15, no. 7 (Jul 2006): 885–96.

Banque mondiale. "Dépenses militaires (% du PIB)." http://donnees.banquemondiale.org/indicateur/MS.MIL.XPND.GD.ZS.

Barnby, Joseph M., Neil W. Bailey, Richard Chambers, and Paul B. Fitzgerald. "How similar are the changes in neural activity resulting from mindfulness practice in contrast to spiritual practice?". *Conscious Cogn* 36 (Nov 2015): 219–32.

Bausell, R. Barker, and Brian M. Berman. "Commentary: alternative medicine: is it a reflection of the continued emergence of the biopsychosocial paradigm?". *American journal of medical quality* 17, no. 1 (Jan-Feb 2002): 28–32.

Bayard, Florence. *L'art de bien mourir au XVe siècle.* Paris: Presses de l'Université de Paris-Sorbonne, 1999.

https://doi.org/10.1515/9783110638950-013

Beauchamp, Tom L., and James F. Childress. *Principles of Biomedical Ethics*. 7th ed. Oxford: Oxford University Press, 2012.

Benaroyo, Lazare. "Éthique et herméneutique du soin." In *La philosophie du soin Éthique, médecine et société*, edited by Lazare Benaroyo, Céline Lefève, Jean-Christophe Mino and Frédérique Worms, 317. Paris: Presses universitaires de France, 2010.

Benning, Tony B. "Limitations of the biopsychosocial model in psychiatry." *Advances in medical education and practice* 6 (2015): 347–52.

Berman, Elisheva, Jon F. Merz, Michael Rudnick, Richard W. Snyder, Katherine K. Rogers, James Lee, and Joshua H. Lipschutz. "Religiosity in a hemodialysis population and its relationship to satisfaction with medical care, satisfaction with life, and adherence." *American Journal of Kidney Diseases* 44, no. 3 (2004): 488–97.

Bernard, Claude. *Principes de médecine expérimentale*. Paris: Quadrige/Presses universitaires de France, 2008 [1947].

Bézy, Olivier. "Quelques commentaires à propos de la célèbre formule de René Leriche: 'La santé c'est la vie dans le silence des organes'." *La revue lacanienne*, no. 3 (2009): 47–50.

Bircher, Johannes. "Towards a Dynamic Definition of Health and Disease." *Medicine, Health Care and Philosophy* 8 (2005): 335–41.

Bjarnason, Dana. "Nursing, religiosity, and end-of-life care: interconnections and implications." *Nursing Clinics of North America* 44, no. 4 (Dec 2009): 517–25.

Boero, Maria E., M. L. Caviglia, R. Monteverdi, Vanda Braida, María Fabello, and Laura M. Zorzella. "Spirituality of health workers: a descriptive study." *Int J Nurs Stud* 42, no. 8 (Nov 2005): 915–21.

Borneman, Tami, Betty Ferrell, and Christina M. Puchalski. "Evaluation of the FICA Tool for Spiritual Assessment." *J Pain Symptom Manage* 40, no. 2 (Aug 2010): 163–73.

Brandt, Pierre-Yves. "L'accompagnement spirituel en milieu hospitalier exige-t-il des compétences spécifiques?". In *Spiritualité en milieu hospitalier*, edited by Pierre-Yves Brandt and Jacques Besson, 15–34. Genève: Labor et Fides, 2015.

Brandt, Pierre-Yves. "La spiritualité: réponse à un besoin, à une soif ou à une quête?". Chap. 2 In *Besoins spirituels: soins, désir, responsabilités*, edited by Eckhard Frick, Dominique Jacquemin and Cosette Odier, 17–31. Bruxelles: Lumen vitae, 2016.

Buchter, Serena, Michel Fontaine, Catherine Piguet, and Brigitte Duc (collaboration). "Du besoin au désir. La dimension spirituelle dans les soins infirmiers: le point de vue infirmier." In *Besoins spirituels Soin, désir, responsabilités*, edited by Dominique Jacquemin, 33–52. Bruxelles: Lumen vitae, 2016.

Büssing, Arndt, Annina Janko, Klaus Baumann, Niels C. Hvidt, and Andreas Kopf. "Spiritual needs among patients with chronic pain diseases and cancer living in a secular society." *Pain Medicine* 14, no. 9 (Sep 2013): 1362–73.

Büssing, Arndt, Sat B. Khalsa, Andreas Michalsen, Karen J. Sherman, and Shirley Telles. "Yoga as a therapeutic intervention." *Evid Based Complement Alternat Med* 2012 (2012): 174291.

Büssing, Arndt, Andreas Michalsen, Hans-Joachim Balzat, Ralf A. Grünther, Thomas Ostermann, Edmund A. Neugebauer, and Peter F. Matthiessen. "Are spirituality and religiosity resources for patients with chronic pain conditions?". *Pain Medicine* 10, no. 2 (Mar 2009): 327–39.

Cahill, Lisa S. "Bioethics, theology, and social change." *J Relig Ethics* 31, no. 3 (Winter 2003): 363–98.

Camargos, Mayara G., Carlos E. Paiva, Eliane M. Barroso, Estela Cristina Carneseca, and Bianca S. R. Paiva. "Understanding the Differences Between Oncology Patients and Oncology Health Professionals Concerning Spirituality/Religiosity: A Cross-Sectional Study." *Medicine* (Baltimore) 94, no. 47 (Nov 2015): e2145.

Campbell, Alastair V. "Secularised bioethics and the passion of religion." *New Rev Bioeth* 1, no. 1 (Nov 2003): 117–26.

Canguilhem, Georges. *Le normal et le pathologique.* Paris: Quadrige/Presses universitaires de France, 1966.

Caputo, John D. *The Weakness of God. A Theology of the Event.* Indiana Series in the Philosophy of Religion. Edited by Merod Westhal. Bloomington: Indiana University Press, 2006.

Caputo, John D. *The Insistence of God. A Theology of Perhaps.* Indiana Series in the Philosophy of Religion. Edited by Merod Westhal. Bloomington: Indiana University Press, 2013.

Caputo, John D. *Truth.* New York: Penguin Books, 2013.

Carson, Ronald A. "Engaged humanities: moral work in the precincts of medicine." *Perspect Biol Med* 50, no. 3 (Summer 2007): 321–33.

Castra, Michel. *Bien mourir. Sociologie des soins palliatifs.* Le Lien social. Edited by Serbe Paugam. Paris: Presses universitaires de France, 2003.

Cavaliere, Terri A., Barbara Daly, Donna Dowling, and Kathleen Montgomery. "Moral distress in neonatal intensive care unit RNs." *Adv Neonatal Care* 10, no. 3 (Jun 2010): 145–56.

Charon, Rita. *Narrative medicine: honoring the stories of illness.* New York: Oxford University Press, 2008.

Châtel, Tanguy. "Les nouvelles cultures de l'accompagnement: les soins palliatifs, une voie 'spirituelle' dans une société de performance." École Pratique des Hautes Études, 2008.

Châtel, Tanguy. *Vivants jusqu'à la mort. Accompagner la souffrance spirituelle en fin de vie.* Paris: Albin Michel, 2013.

Cheatle, Martin D. "Biopsychosocial Approach to Assessing and Managing Patients with Chronic Pain." *The Medical Clinics of North America* 100, no. 1 (Jan 2016): 43–53.

Cherblanc, Jacques, and Guy Jobin. "Vers une psychologisation du religieux ? Le cas des institutions sanitaires au Québec." *Archives de sciences sociales des religions* 163, no. 3 (2013): 39–62.

Chochinov, Harvey Max. "Dignity Therapy: A Novel Psychotherapeutic Intervention for Patients near the End of Life." *Journal of Clinical Oncology* 23, no. 4 (2005): 5520–25.

Chochinov, Harvey Max. "Dying, Dignity, and New Horizons in Palliative End-of-Life Care." *CA A Cancer Journal for the Clinicians* 56 (2006): 84–103.

Chochinov, Harvey Max. "Dignity and the essence of medicine: the A, B, C, and D of dignity conserving care." *Bmj* 335, no. 7612 (Jul 28 2007): 184–7.

Chochinov, Harvey Max. "Dignity-Based Approaches in the Care of Terminally Ill Patients." *Current Opinion in Supportive and Palliative Care* 2 (2008): 49–53.

Chochinov, Harvey Max, Thomas Hassard, Susan McClement, Thomas Hack, Linda J. Kristjanson, Mike Harlos, Shane Sinclair, and Alison Murray. "The patient dignity inventory: a novel way of measuring dignity-related distress in palliative care." *J Pain Symptom Manage* 36, no. 6 (Dec 2008): 559–71.

Chochinov, Harvey Max, Linda J. Kristjanson, William Breitbart, Susan McClement, Thomas F. Hack, Thomas Hassard, and Mike Harlos. "Effect of dignity therapy on distress and end-of-life experience in terminally ill patients: a randomised controlled trial." *Lancet Oncol* 12, no. 8 (Aug 2011): 753–62.

Clark, David. "From Margins to Center: A Review of the History of Palliative Care in Cancer." *The Lancet*, no. 8 (2007): 430–38.

Clements, Andrea D., Tifani R. Fletcher, Natalie A. Cyphers, Anna V. Ermakova, and Beth Bailey. "RSAS-3: validation of a very brief measure of Religious Commitment for use in health research." *J Relig Health* 54, no. 1 (Feb 2015): 134–52.

Connor, Stephen R. "Development of hospice and palliative care in the United States." *Omega* (Westport) 56, no. 1 (2007): 89–99.

Copley, Terence. *Spiritual development in the State school: a perspective on worship and spirituality in the education system of England and Wales.* Exeter: University of Exeter Press, 2000.

Cotton, Sian, Christina M. Puchalski, Susan N. Sherman, Joseph M. Mrus, Amy H. Peterman, Judith Feinberg, Kenneth I. Pargament, Amy C. Justice, Alan C. Leonard, and Joel Tsevat. "Spirituality and religion in patients with HIV/AIDS." *J Gen Intern Med* 21 Suppl 5 (Dec 2006): S5–13.

Craigie, Frederic C., Jr. "Weaving spirituality into organizational life. Suggestions for processes and programs." *Health Prog* 79, no. 2 (Mar-Apr 1998): 25–8, 32.

Craven, Ruth F., and Constance J. Hirnle. *Fundamentals of nursing: human health and function.* 5th ed. Philadelphia: Lippincott Williams & Wilkins, 2007.

Crenshaw, James L. "Wisdom Literature." In *The Oxford Companion to the Bible*, edited by Bruce M. Metzger and Michael D. Coogan. New York: Oxford University Press, 1993.

Crescentini, Cristiano, Salvatore M. Aglioti, Franco Fabbro, and Cosimo Urgesi. "Virtual lesions of the inferior parietal cortex induce fast changes of implicit religiousness/spirituality." *Cortex* 54 (May 2014): 1–15.

D'Aquili, Eugene G., and Andrew B. Newberg. *The mystical mind: probing the biology of religious experience.* Minneapolis, MN: Fortress Press, 1999.

Daaleman, Timothy P., and Bruce B. Frey. "The Spirituality Index of Well-Being: a new instrument for health-related quality-of-life research." *Annals Of Family Medicine* 2, no. 5 (2004): 499–503.

Dante, Alighieri. *La divine comédie: le paradis = [paradisio]: texte original.* Translated by Jacqueline Risset. Paris: Flammarion, 1992.

Davison, Sara N., and Gian S. Jhangri. "Existential and religious dimensions of spirituality and their relationship with health-related quality of life in chronic kidney disease." *Clinical Journal of the American Society of Nephrology* 5, no. 11 (Nov 2010): 1969–76.

Davison, Sara N., and Gian S. Jhangri. "Existential and supportive care needs among patients with chronic kidney disease." *J Pain Symptom Manage* 40, no. 6 (Dec 2010): 838–43.

Davison, Sara N., and Gian S. Jhangri. "The relationship between spirituality, psychosocial adjustment to illness, and health-related quality of life in patients with advanced chronic kidney disease." *J Pain Symptom Manage* 45, no. 2 (Feb 2013): 170–8.

Dictionnaire de la vie spirituelle. Paris: Cerf, 1983.

de Certeau, Michel. *La fable mystique II. XVIe-XVIIe siècle.* Bibliothèque des histoires. Paris: Gallimard, 2013.

Debnam, Katrina J., Cheryl L. Holt, Eddie M. Clark, David L. Roth, Herman R. Foushee, Martha Crowther, Mona Fouad, and Penny L. Southward. "Spiritual health locus of control and health behaviors in African Americans." *Am J Health Behav* 36, no. 3 (Mar 2012): 360–72.

Dell'Oro, Roberto. "Theological discourse and the postmodern condition: the case of bioethics." *Med Health Care Philos* 5, no. 2 (2002): 127–36.

Dent, Nicolas. "Vertu. Éthique de la vertu." In *Dictionnaire d'éthique et de philosophie morale*, edited by Monique Canto-Sperber, 2011–19. Paris: Quadrige/Presses universitaires de France, 2004.

Department for children schools and families. *Religious education in English schools: Non-statutory guidance 2010*. Government of United Kingdom, 2010. https://www.gov.uk/government/uploads/system/uploads/attachment_data/file/190260/DCSF-00114–2010.pdf.

Desbiens, Jean-F., and Lise Fillion. "Coping strategies, emotional outcomes and spiritual quality of life in palliative care nurses." *Int J Palliat Nurs* 13, no. 6 (Jun 2007): 291–300.

Dos Anjos, Marcio F., and Hubert F. Lepargneur. "Bioethics and Christian theology in Brazil." *J Int Bioethique* 19, no. 1–2 (Mar-Jun 2008): 43–53, 194–5.

Douglass, Laura. "Thinking through the body: the conceptualization of yoga as therapy for individuals with eating disorders." *Eat Disord* 19, no. 1 (Jan-Feb 2011): 83–96.

Doyle, Derek. "Palliative medicine in Britain." *Omega* (Westport) 56, no. 1 (2007): 77–88.

Duggleby, Wendy, Dan Cooper, and Kelly Penz. "Hope, self-efficacy, spiritual well-being and job satisfaction." *J Adv Nurs* 65, no. 11 (Nov 2009): 2376–85.

Ehrenberg, Alain. *La fatigue d'être soi: dépression et société*. Paris: O. Jacob, 1998.

Ehrenberg, Alain. *La société du malaise*. Paris: Odile Jacob, 2010.

Engel, George L. "The need for a new medical model: a challenge for biomedicine." *Science* 196, no. 4286 (1977): 129–36.

Engel, George L. "How much longer must medicine's science be bound by a seventeenth century world view?". *Psychotherapy and psychosomatics* 57, no. 1–2 (1992): 3–16.

Engel, George L. "From biomedical to biopsychosocial. 1. Being scientific in the human domain." *Psychotherapy and psychosomatics* 66, no. 2 (1997): 57–62.

Engel, George L. "From biomedical to biopsychosocial. Being scientific in the human domain." *Psychosomatics* 38, no. 6 (Nov-Dec 1997): 521–8.

Érasme. *La préparation à la mort*. Montréal: Éditions Paulines/Apostolat des Éditions, 1976[1533].

Fava, Giovanni A., and Nicoletta Sonino. "The biopsychosocial model thirty years later." *Psychotherapy and psychosomatics* 77, no. 1 (2008): 1–2.

Feuille, Margaret, and Kenneth I. Pargament. "Pain, mindfulness, and spirituality: A randomized controlled trial comparing effects of mindfulness and relaxation on pain-related outcomes in migraineurs." *Journal of Health Psychology* 20, no. 8 (Aug 2015): 1090–106.

Fischbeck, Sabine, Bernd-O. Maier, Ulrike Reinholz, Cornelia Nehring, Rainer Schwab, Manfred E. Beutel, and Martin Weber. "Assessing somatic, psychosocial, and spiritual distress of patients with advanced cancer: development of the Advanced Cancer Patients' Distress Scale." *Am J Hosp Palliat Care* 30, no. 4 (Jun 2013): 339–46.

Fitzpatrick, Scott J., Ian H. Kerridge, Christopher F. C. Jordens, Laurie Zoloth, Christopher Tollefsen, Karma L. Tsomo, Michael P. Jensen, Abdulaziz Sachedina, and Deepak Sarma. "Religious Perspectives on Human Suffering: Implications for Medicine and Bioethics." *J Relig Health* 55, no. 1 (Feb 2016): 159–73.

Foucault, Michel. *Naissance de la clinique.* 6th ed. Paris: Quadrige/Presses universitaires de France, 2000 [1963].

Frank, Arthur W. *The Wounded Storyteller. Body, Illness, and Ethics.* Chicago: The University of Chicago Press, 1995.

Frank, Arthur W. *Letting stories breathe: a socio-narratology.* Chicago: University of Chicago Press, 2010.

Freedman, Alfred M. "The biopsychosocial paradigm and the future of psychiatry." *Comprehensive psychiatry* 36, no. 6 (Nov-Dec 1995): 397–406.

Frick, Eckhard, Carola Riedner, Martin J. Fegg, Silke Hauf, and Gian D. Borasio. "A clinical interview assessing cancer patients' spiritual needs and preferences." *European Journal of Cancer Care* 15, no. 3 (2006): 238–43.

Fukui, Sadaaki, Vincent R. Starnino, and Holly B. Nelson-Becker. "Spiritual well-being of people with psychiatric disabilities: the role of religious attendance, social network size and sense of control." *Community Ment Health J* 48, no. 2 (Apr 2012): 202–11.

Fuller, Robert C. *Spiritual, but not religious understanding unchurched America.* Oxford: Oxford University Press, 2001. http://dx.doi.org/10.1093/0195146808.001.0001.

Gadamer, Hans-Georg. *Vérité et méthode. Les grandes lignes d'une herméneutique philosophique.* L'ordre philosophique. Edited by Alain Badiou and Barbara Cassin. Paris: Seuil, 1996 [1960].

Gagnon, Pierre, Lise Fillion, Michèle Girard, François Tardif, and Marie-Anik Robitaille. "Le rôle central des questions existentielles et spirituelles en oncologie et en soins palliatifs." In *Spiritualités et biomédecine Enjeux d'une intégration*, edited by Guy Jobin, Jean-Marc Charron and Michel Nyabenda, 115–32. Québec: Presses de l'Université Laval, 2013.

Garschagen, Alexander, Monique A. H. Steegers, Alfonsus van Bergen, Johannes Jochijms, Titus Skrabanja, Hubertus Vrijhoef, Rob Smeets, and Kris Vissers. "Is There a Need for Including Spiritual Care in Interdisciplinary Rehabilitation of Chronic Pain Patients? Investigating an Innovative Strategy." *Pain Practice* 15, no. 7 (Sep 2015): 671–87.

Gauchet, Marcel. *Le désenchantement du monde: une histoire politique de la religion.* Paris: Gallimard, 1985.

"The Goals of Medicine: Setting New Priorities. Special Supplement." *The Hastings Center Report* 26, no. 6 (1996): S1–S27.

Godelier, Maurice. "Maladie et santé selon les sociétés et les cultures." In *Maladie et santé selon les sociétés et les cultures*, edited by Jean-Pierre Dozon, Sylvie Fainzang, Maurice Godelier, Elisabeth Hsu and Francis Zimmermann, 13–29. Paris: Presses universitaires de France, 2011.

Gomi, Sachiko, Vincent R. Starnino, and Edward R. Canda. "Spiritual assessment in mental health recovery." *Community Mental Health Journal* 50, no. 4 (2014): 447–53.

Gouvernement du Québec. *Education Act.* http://www.legisquebec.gouv.qc.ca/en/ShowDoc/cs/I-13.3.

Gouvernement du Québec. "Loi sur les services de santé et les services sociaux." In *S-42*, edited by Ministère de la santé et des services sociaux. Québec: Gouvernement du Québec, 2005.

Gouvernement du Québec. "S-4.2 Loi sur les services de santé et les services sociaux." edited by Ministère de la santé et des services sociaux. Québec: Gouvernement du Québec, 2005.

Greenberg, Jonathan, Benjamin G. Shapero, David Mischoulon, and Sara W. Lazar. "Mindfulness-based cognitive therapy for depressed individuals improves suppression of irrelevant mental-sets." *Eur Arch Psychiatry Clin Neurosci* 267, no. 3 (Apr 2017): 277–82.

Gregg, Godfrey. "I'm a Jesus girl: coping stories of Black American women diagnosed with breast cancer." *J Relig Health* 50, no. 4 (Dec 2011): 1040–53.

Greisch, Jean. *L'âge herméneutique de la raison*. Paris: Éditions du Cerf, 1985.

Habermas, Jürgen. "De l'usage pragmatique, éthique et moral de la raison pratique." Translated by Mark Hunyadi. In *De l'éthique de la discussion*, edited by Jürgen Habermas. Champs, 95–110. Paris: Flammarion, 1992.

Häring, Bernard. *Medical Ethics*. Notre Dame, Ind.: Fides, 1973.

Heelas, Paul. *Spiritualities of Life. New Age Romanticism and Consumptive Capitalism*. Religion and Spirituality in the Modern World. Edited by Paul Heelas and Linda Woodhead. Oxford: Blackwell, 2008.

Heelas, Paul, and Linda Woodhead. *The spiritual revolution: why religion is giving way to spirituality*. Malden, MA: Blackwell Pub, 2005.

Henderson, Virginia. *Les principes fondamentaux des soins infirmiers du CII*. Genève: Conseil international des infirmières (CII), 2003 [1960].

Herring, Malcolm B., and Jon D. Rahman. "Physicians and spirituality. St. Vincent Indianapolis has a program that encourages spiritual development in doctors." *Health Prog* 85, no. 4 (Jul-Aug 2004): 43–7.

Hornborg, Anne-C. "Designing rites to re-enchant secularized society: new varieties of spiritualized therapy in contemporary Sweden." *J Relig Health* 51, no. 2 (Jun 2012): 402–18.

Hougaard, Anders, Ulrich Lindberg, Nanna Arngrim, Henrik B. W. Larsson, Jes Olesen, Faisal M. Amin, Messoud Ashina, and Brian T. Haddock. "Evidence of a Christmas spirit network in the brain: functional MRI study." *Bmj* 351 (Dec 16 2015): h6266.

Hume, Rosemary, Sharon Richardt, and Beth Applegate. "Spirituality and work. Indianapolis's Seton Cove Center seeks to integrate spirituality into the workplace." *Health Prog* 84, no. 3 (May-Jun 2003): 20–5.

Imber, Jonathan B., ed. *Therapeutic Culture. Triumph and Defeat*. Herndon, VA: Transaction, 2004.

International, Association for the Study of Pain. "IASP Taxonomy." International Association for the Study of Pain, http://www.iasp-pain.org/Education/Content.aspx?ItemNumber=1698&navItemNumber=576.

Jacquemin, Dominique. *La bioéthique et la question de Dieu: une voie séculière d'intériorité et de spiritualité?* Montréal: Médiaspaul, 1996.

Jacquemin, Dominique. *Bioéthique, médecine et souffrance: jalons pour une théologie de l'échec*. Montréal: Médiaspaul, 2002.

Jacquemin, Dominique. "La confrontation avec la souffrance: un lieu pour penser le lien entre éthique et spiritualité." In *Spiritualité: interpellation et enjeux pour le soin et la médecine*, edited by Danièle Leboul and Dominique Jacquemin. Les carnets de l'espace éthique de Bretagne occidentale, 53–78. Montpellier: Sauramps médical, 2010.

Jacquemin, Dominique. *Quand l'autre souffre. Éthique et spiritualité.* Donner raison. Bruxelles: Lessius, 2010.

Jacquemin, Dominique, ed. *Besoins spirituels. Soins, désir, responsabilités.* Edited by Eckhard Frick, Dominique Jacquemin and Cosette Odier Vol. 7, Soins et spiritualités. Bruxelles: Lumen vitae, 2016.

Jobin, Guy. "Quand narrer, c'est (re)construire: intrigue et récit en temps de maladie." In *L'intrigue dans le récit biblique*, edited by Anne Pasquier, Daniel Marguerat and André Wénin. Bibliotheca Ephemeridum Theologicarum Lovaniensis, 237, 87–107. Leuven: Peeters, 2010.

Jobin, Guy. "La spiritualité: facteur de résistance au pouvoir biomédical de soigner ?". *Revue d'éthique et de théologie morale* 266, no. HS (2011): 131–49.

Jobin, Guy. *Des religions à la spiritualité: une appropriation biomédicale du religieux dans l'hôpital.* Bruxelles: Lumen vitae, 2012.

Jobin, Guy. "Êtes-vous en belle santé? Sur l'esthétisation de la spiritualité en biomédecine." Chap. 3 In *Spiritualités et biomédecine Enjeux d'une intégration*, edited by Guy Jobin, Jean-Marc Charron and Michel Nyabenda, 41–61. Québec: Presses de l'Université Laval, 2013.

Jobin, Guy. *Des religions à la spiritualité. Une appropriation biomédicale du religieux dans l'hôpital.* Soins et spiritualités. Edited by Eckhard Frick and Cosette Odier. 2nd ed. Bruxelles: Lumen vitae, 2013[2012].

Jobin, Guy. "Santé, bien-être et spiritualité: une évaluation critique." *Interaçoes – Cultura E Comunidade* 11, no. 20 (2016): 31–47.

Jobin, Guy. "Development of the Connection Between Spirituality and Medicine: Historical and Current Issues in Clinics." *Spiritual Care* 6, no. 2 (2017): 1–8.

Jobin, Guy. "Quelle anthropologie pour inclure la dimension spirituelle aux soins? Perspectives d'avenir." *Revue théologique de Louvain* 48, no. 4 (2017): 510–34.

Jobin, Guy. "La prise en compte de l'expérience spirituelle en soins palliatifs: un cas de mutation des représentations de la spiritualité." *Laval théologique et philosophique* 72, no. 3 (octobre 2016): 449–63.

Jobin, Guy, Anne C. Guyon, Maxime Allard, Didier Caenepeel, Jacques Cherblanc, Johanne Lessard, and Nicolas Vonarx. "Spirituality, according to palliative caregivers. A systemic Analysis (Wie Spiritualität in Palliative Care verstanden wird. Eine Systemische Analyse." *Spiritual Care* 2, no. 1 (2013): 17–26.

Jobin, Guy, Anne C. Guyon, Maxime Allard, Didier Caenepeel, Jacques Cherblanc, and Nicolas Vonarx. "Bénévolat et spiritualité en soins palliatifs." Chap. 15 In *Le bénévolat en soins palliatifs ou l'art d'accompagner*, edited by Andrée Sévigny, Manon Champagne and Manal Guirguis-Younger, 275–92. Québec: Maison Michel Sarrazin/Presses de l'Université Laval, 2013.

Kabat-Zinn, Jon. *Au coeur de la tourmente, la pleine conscience.* Bien-être. Edited by Ahmed Djouder. Paris: Éditions J'ai lu, 2009[1990].

Karl, Suzanne R., and Jimmie C. Holland. "The Roots of Psychosomatic Medicine II: George L. Engel." *Psychosomatics* 56, no. 6 (Nov-Dec 2015): 630–3.

Kaur, Devinder, Murali Sambasivan, and Naresh Kumar. "Effect of spiritual intelligence, emotional intelligence, psychological ownership and burnout on caring behaviour of nurses: a cross-sectional study." *J Clin Nurs* 22, no. 21–22 (Nov 2013): 3192–202.

Kim, Jeong-H., Young-D. Son, Jong-H. Kim, Eun-J. Choi, Sang-Y. Lee, Yo-H. Joo, Young-B. Kim, and Zang-H. Cho. "Self-transcendence trait and its relationship with in vivo serotonin transporter availability in brainstem raphe nuclei: An ultra-high resolution PET-MRI study." *Brain Res* 1629 (Dec 10 2015): 63–71.

Kimmel, Paul L., Seth L. Emont, John M. Newmann, Helen Danko, and Alvin H. Moss. "ESRD patient quality of life: symptoms, spiritual beliefs, psychosocial factors, and ethnicity." *American Journal of Kidney Diseases* 42, no. 4 (Oct 2003): 713–21.

Ko, Benjamin, Amandeep Khurana, Judy Spencer, Barbara Scott, Marsha Hahn, and Mary Hammes. "Religious beliefs and quality of life in an American inner-city haemodialysis population." *Nephrology Dialysis Transplant* 22, no. 10 (Oct 2007): 2985–90.

Koenig, Harold G. "Religion, spirituality, and health: the research and clinical implications." *ISRN Psychiatry* (2012): 278730.

Koenig, Harold G., Verna Benner Carson, and Dana E. King. *Handbook of religion and health.* 2nd ed. Oxford: Oxford University Press, 2012.

Kontos, Nicholas. "Perspective: biomedicine–menace or straw man? Reexamining the biopsychosocial argument." *Academic Medicine* 86, no. 4 (Apr 2011): 509–15.

Korzinski, David. "A spectrum of spirituality: Canadians keep the faith to varying degrees, but few reject it entirely." Angus Reid Institute, http://angusreid.org/religion-in-canada-150/.

Kreitzer, Mary Jo, Cynthia R. Gross, On-anong Waleekhachonloet, Maryanne Reilly-Spong, and Marcia Byrd. "The Brief Serenity Scale: A Psychometric Analysis of a Measure of Spirituality and Well-Being." *Journal of Holistic Nursing* 27, no. 1 (March 1, 2009 2009): 7–16.

Lafont, Ghislain. *La sagesse et la prophétie. Modèles théologiques.* Paris: Cerf, 1999.

Lafontaine, Céline. *La société post-mortelle: la mort, l'individu et le lien social à l'ère des technosciences.* Paris: Seuil, 2008.

Lamau, Marie-Louise, and Lucie Hacpille. "Origine et inspiration." Chap. 1 In *Manuel de soins palliatifs*, edited by Dominique Jacquemin and Didier de Broucker, 9–33. Paris: Dunod, 2009.

Larchet, Jean-Claude. *Thérapeutique des maladies spirituelles.* l'Arbre de Jessé. 2 vols. Vol. 1, Paris: Éditions de l'Ancre, 1991.

Larson, Gerald James, and Ram S. Bhattacharya. *Yoga: India's philosophy of meditation.* 1st ed. Delhi: Motilal Banarsidass Publishers, 2008.

Latour, Bruno. *Pandora's Hope. Essays on the Reality of Science Studies.* Cambridge Ma.: Harvard University Press, 1999.

Legault, Georges-A. *Professionnalisme et délibération éthique.* Québec: Presses de l'Université du Québec, 2007.

Lemieux, Raymond. "La dialectique de la communauté et du réseau dans le champ religieux." In *Communautés et socialités Formes et force du lien social dans la modernité tardive*, edited by Francine Saillant and Éric Gagnon, 75–94. Montréal: Liber, 2005.

Leplège, Alain, and Sylvie Duverger. "Qualité de la vie." In *Dictionnaire d'éthique et de philosophie morale*, edited by Monique Canto-Sperber, 1601–05. Paris: Quadrige/Presses universitaires de France, [1996] 2004.

Letourneau, Jim. "Mission Integration and Workplace Spirituality." *Health Prog* 97, no. 2 (Mar-Apr 2016): 30–2.

Libera, Alain de. *Penser au Moyen Âge*. Paris: Seuil, 1991.

Liogier, Raphaël. *Souci de soi, conscience du monde: vers une religion globale? [Concern for Oneself, Concern for the World. Toward a Global Religion?]*. Paris: Armand Colin, 2012.

Loiselle, Carmen G., and Michelle M. Sterling. "Views on death and dying among health care workers in an Indian cancer care hospice: balancing individual and collective perspectives." *Palliat Med* 26, no. 3 (Apr 2012): 250–6.

Louie, Lila. "The effectiveness of yoga for depression: a critical literature review." *Issues Ment Health Nurs* 35, no. 4 (Apr 2014): 265–76.

Lowis, Michael J., Anthony C. Edwards, and Mary Burton. "Coping with retirement: well-being, health, and religion." *J Psychol* 143, no. 4 (Jul 2009): 427–48.

Luckmann, Thomas. *The Invisible Religion. The Problem of Religion in Modern Society*. New York: MacMillan, 1967.

Mauss, Marcel. "Essai sur le don. Forme et raison de l'échange dans les sociétés archaïques." In *Sociologie et anthropologie*, edited by Marcel Mauss, 143–279. Paris: Quadrige/Presses universitaires de France, 2004[1950].

McCrae, Niall, and Rob Whitley. "Exaltation in Temporal Lobe Epilepsy: Neuropsychiatric Symptom or Portal to the Divine?". *Journal of Medical Humanities* 35, no. 3 (2014): 241–55.

McCullough, Michael E., and Brian L. Willoughby. "Religion, self-regulation, and self-control: Associations, explanations, and implications." *Psychol Bull* 135, no. 1 (Jan 2009): 69–93.

McGuire, Maureen. "Toward workplace spirituality. St. Louis-based Ascension Health is attending to the "spirit in work"." *Health Prog* 85, no. 6 (Nov-Dec 2004): 14–6.

Meyer, Philippe. *Philosophie de la médecine*. Paris: Bernard Grasset, 2000.

Mitroff, Ian I., and Elizabeth A. Denton. *A spiritual audit of corporate America: a hard look at spirituality, religion, and values in the workplace*. 1st ed. San Francisco: Jossey-Bass Publishers, 1999.

Mohr, Sylvia, Christiane Gillieron, Laurence Borras, Pierre-Yves Brandt, and Philippe Huguelet. "The assessment of spirituality and religiousness in schizophrenia." *Journal of Nervous and Mental Disease*, no. 195 (2007): 247–53.

Monod-Zorzi, Stéfanie. *Soins aux personnes âgées. Intégrer la spiritualité?* Soins et spiritualités. Edited by Eckhard Frick and Cosette Odier. Vol. 2, Bruxelles: Lumen vitae, 2012.

Monod-Zorzi, Stéfanie, Estelle Martin, Brenda Spencer, Étienne Rochat, and Christophe Büla. "Validation of the Spiritual Distress Assessment Tool in older hospitalized patients." *BMC Geriatr* 12 (2012): 13.

Monod, Stéfanie M., Étienne Rochat, Christophe J. Büla, Guy Jobin, Estelle Martin, and Brenda Spencer. "The spiritual distress assessment tool: an instrument to assess spiritual distress in hospitalised elderly persons." *BMC Geriatr* 10 (2010): 88.

Moreira-Almeida, Alexander, and Harold G. Koenig. "Religiousness and spirituality in fibromyalgia and chronic pain patients." *Current Pain and Headache Reports* 12, no. 5 (Oct 2008): 327–32.

Müller, Denis. "Tragique." In *Dictionnaire encyclopédique d'éthique chrétienne*, edited by Laurent Lemoine, Eric Gaziaux and Denis Müller. Paris: Cerf, 2013.

Murray, Ruth Beckmann, and Judith Proctor Zentner. *Nursing Concepts for Health Promotion.* London: Prentice Hall, 1989.

Murray, Ruth Beckmann, Judith Proctor Zentner, and Richard Yakimo. "Spiritual and Religious Influences." Chap. 7 In *Health Promotion Strategies Through the Life Span*, 181–211. Upper Saddle River, NJ: Pearson/Prentice Hall, 2009.

Nadeau, Gilles. "Le coeur s'agrandit." Chap. 14 In *Le bénévolat en soins palliatifs ou l'art d'accompagner*, edited by Andrée Sévigny, Manon Champagne and Manal Guirguis-Younger, 257–73. Québec: Maison Michel-Sarrazin/Presses de l'Université Laval, 2013.

Nader, Mélissa. "La médicalisation: concept, phénomène et processus. Émergence, diffusion et reconfigurations des usages du terme médicalisation dans la littérature sociologique." Université du Québec à Montréal, 2012.

NANDA International. "Détresse spirituelle." In *Diagnostics infirmiers Définitions et classification 2012–2014*, 439. Issy-les-Moulineaux: Elsevier Masson, 2013.

NANDA International. "Motivation à améliorer son bien-être spirituel." In *Diagnostics infirmiers Définitions et classification 2012–2014*, 434. Issy-les-Moulineaux: Elsevier Masson, 2013.

Nandram, Sharda S., and Margot Esther Borden. *Spirituality and business exploring possibilities for a new management paradigm.* Berlin: Springer, 2010. http://dx.doi.org/10.1007/978-3-642-02661-4.

Newberg, Andre B., and Mark Robert Waldman. *Words can change your brain: 12 conversation strategies to build trust, resolve conflict, and increase intimacy.* New York: Plume, 2013.

Newberg, Andrew B. *Principles of neurotheology.* Farnham, Surrey, England: Ashgate Pub, 2010.

Newberg, Andrew B., Eugene G. D'Aquili, and Vince Rause. *Why God won't go away: brain science and the biology of belief.* 1st ed. New York: Ballantine Books, 2001.

Newberg, Andrew B., Eugene G. D'Aquili, and Vince Rause. *Pourquoi "Dieu" ne disparaîtra pas: quand la science explique la religion.* Vannes: Sully, 2003.

Newberg, Andrew B., and Mark Robert Waldman. *Why we believe what we believe: uncovering our biological need for meaning, spirituality, and truth.* New York: Free Press, 2006.

OCDE. "Statistiques de l'OCDE sur la santé 2016." http://oecd.org/fr/els/systemes-sante/base-donnees-sante.htm.

Oser, Fritz, and Paul Gmünder. *L'homme, son développement religieux. Étude de structuralisme génétique.* Translated by Louis Ridez. Sciences humaines et religions. Paris: Cerf, 1991[1988].

Parsons, Talcott. *The Social System.* New York: The Free Press, 1951.

Patel, Samir S., Viral S. Shah, Rolf A. Peterson, and Paul L. Kimmel. "Psychosocial variables, quality of life, and religious beliefs in ESRD patients treated with hemodialysis." *American Journal of Kidney Diseases* 40, no. 5 (Nov 2002): 1013–22.

Pauchant, Thierry C., and Le Forum international sur le management l'éthique et la spiritualité. *Pour un management éthique et spirituel: défis, cas, outils et questions.* Saint-Laurent, Québec: Fides, 2000.

Pauchant, Thierry C., and Le Forum international sur le management l'éthique et la spiritualité. *Ethics and spirituality at work: hopes and pitfalls of the search for meaning in organizations.* Westport, Conn: Quorum Books, 2002.

Pellegrino, Edmund D., John Langan, and John Collins Harvey. *Catholic perspectives on medical morals: foundational issues.* Dordrecht: Kluwer Academic Publishers, 1989.

Pellegrino, Edmund D., and David C. Thomasma. *For the patient's good: the restoration of beneficence in health care.* New York: Oxford University Press, 1988.

Peterman, Amy H., George Fitchett, Marianne J. Brady, Lesbia Hernandez, and David Cella. "Measuring spiritual well-being in people with cancer: the functional assessment of chronic illness therapy—Spiritual Well-being Scale (FACIT-Sp)." *Ann Behav Med* 24, no. 1 (Winter 2002): 49–58.

Peterman, Amy H., Charlie L. Reeve, Eboni C. Winford, Sian Cotton, John M. Salsman, Richard McQuellon, Joel Tsevat, and Cassie Campbell. "Measuring meaning and peace with the FACIT-spiritual well-being scale: distinction without a difference?". *Psychol Assess* 26, no. 1 (Mar 2014): 127–37.

Pigeaud, Jackie. "L'esthétique de Galien." *Mètis Anthropologie des mondes grecs anciens* 6, no. 1–2 (1991): 7–42.

Pigeaud, Jackie. *L'art et le vivant. nrf essais.* Paris: Gallimard, 1995.

Pigeaud, Jackie. *Poétiques du corps. Aux origines de la médecine.* Paris: Les Belles Lettres, 2009.

Pirkola, Heidi, Piia Rantakokko, and Marjo Suhonen. "Workplace spirituality in health care: an integrated review of the literature." *J Nurs Manag* 24, no. 7 (May 24 2016): 859–68.

Polzer, Rebecca L., and Margaret S. Miles. "Spirituality in African Americans with diabetes: self-management through a relationship with God." *Qualitative health research* 17, no. 2 (2007): 176–88.

Post, Stephen G., Christina M. Puchalski, and David B. Larson. "Physicians and patient spirituality: professional boundaries, competency, and ethics." *Ann Intern Med* 132, no. 7 (Apr 4 2000): 578–83.

Prigogine, Ilya, and Isabelle Stengers. *La nouvelle alliance: métamorphose de la science.* Paris: Gallimard, 1980.

Puchalski, Christina M. "Formal and informal spiritual assessment." *Asian Pac J Cancer Prev* 11 Suppl 1 (2010): 51–7.

Puchalski, Christina M. "The FICA Spiritual History Tool #274." *J Palliat Med* 17, no. 1 (Jan 2014): 105–6.

Puchalski, Christina M., Benjamin Blatt, and George Handzo. "In reply to Salander and Hamberg." *Academic Medicine* 89, no. 11 (Nov 2014): 1430–1.

Puchalski, Christina M., and Betty Ferrell. *Making Health Care Whole. Integrating Spirituality into Patient Care.* West Conshohocken, Pa: Templeton Press, 2010.

Puchalski, Christina M., David B. Larson, and Stephen G. Post. "Physicians and Patient Spirituality." *Ann Intern Med* 133, no. 9 (Nov 7 2000): 748–49.

Puchalski, Christina M., Beverly Lunsford, Mary H. Harris, and Rabbi T. Miller. "Interdisciplinary spiritual care for seriously ill and dying patients: a collaborative model." *Cancer J* 12, no. 5 (Sep-Oct 2006): 398–416.

Puchalski, Christina M., Stephen G. Post, and Richard P. Sloan. "Physicians and patients' spirituality." *Virtual Mentor* 11, no. 10 (2009): 804–15.

Puchalski, Christina M., and Anna L. Romer. "Taking a Spiritual History Allows Clinicians to Understand Patients More Fully." *Journal of Palliative Medicine* 3, no. 1 (2000/03/01 2000): 129–37.

Pugh, Edwin J., Robert Song, Vicki Whittaker, and John Blenkinsopp. "A profile of the belief system and attitudes to end-of-life decisions of senior clinicians working in a National Health Service Hospital in the United Kingdom." *Palliat Med* 23, no. 2 (Mar 2009): 158–64.

Ramsey, Paul. *The Patient as Person.* New Haven: Yale University Press, 1970.

Rawls, John. *La justice comme équité. Une reformulation de Théorie de la justice.* Montréal: Boréal, 2004.

Redmond, Larry W. "Spiritual coping tools of religious victims of childhood sexual abuse." *J Pastoral Care Counsel* 68, no. 1–2 (Mar-Jun 2014): 3.

Richter, Daniel. "Chronic mental illness and the limits of the biopsychosocial model." *Medicine, health care, and philosophy* 2, no. 1 (1999): 21–30.

Ricœur, Paul. *Amour et justice.* Paris: Éditions Points, 2008.

Ricoeur, Paul. *Temps et récit. T.2 La configuration dans le récit de fiction.* Points Essais, 228. Paris: Seuil, 1984.

Ricoeur, Paul. *Soi-même comme un autre.* Points essais, 330. Paris: Seuil, 1990.

Ricoeur, Paul. "Le concept de responsabilité. Essai d'analyse sémantique." In *Le juste I,* 41–70. Paris: Éditions Esprit, 1995.

Rieff, Philip. *The Triumph of the Therapeutic. Uses of Faith after Freud.* Chicago: University of Chicago Press, 1966.

Ross, Collin A. "Talking about God with Trauma Survivors." *Am J Psychother* 70, no. 4 (Dec 31 2016): 429–37.

Ross, Linda. "Spiritual care in nursing: an overview of the research to date." *Journal of Clinical Nursing* 15, no. 7 (Jul 2006): 852–62.

Rousseau, Jean-Jacques. *Profession de foi du vicaire savoyard.* folio essais. Paris: Gallimard, 1969[1762].

Roy, Louis. *Libérer le désir.* Montréal: Médiaspaul, 2009.

Rushton, Cynda H., Joyce Batcheller, Kaia Schroeder, and Pamela Donohue. "Burnout and Resilience Among Nurses Practicing in High-Intensity Settings." *Am J Crit Care* 24, no. 5 (Sep 2015): 412–20.

Salander, Pär, and Katarina Hamberg. "Why 'Spirituality' Instead of 'The Humanistic Side of Medicine'?". *Academic Medicine* 89, no. 11 (2014): 1430.

Salin, Dominique. *L'expérience spirituelle et son langage: leçons sur la tradition mystique chrétienne.* Paris: Éditions des facultés jésuites de Paris, 2015.

Saracci, Rodolfo. "The World Health Organisation Needs to Reconsider Its Definition of Health." *British Medical Journal* 314, no. 7091 (1997): 1409–10.

Saraga, Micharl, Abraham Fuks, and J. Donald Boudreau. "George Engel's Epistemology of Clinical Practice." *Perspectives in biology and medicine* 57, no. 4 (Autumn 2014): 482–94.

Sasser, Charles G., and Christina M. Puchalski. "The humanistic clinician: traversing the science and art of health care." *J Pain Symptom Manage* 39, no. 5 (May 2010): 936–40.

Saunders, Cicely. "Caring for cancer." *J R Soc Med* 91, no. 8 (Aug 1998): 439–41.

Saunders, David C. "Origins: international perspectives, then and now." *Hosp J* 14, no. 3–4 (1999): 1–7.

Scambler, Graham. "Deviance, Sick Role and Stigma." Chap. 13 In *Sociology as Applied to Medicine*, edited by Graham Scambler, 205–17. Edimbourg: Saunders Elsevier, 2008.

Seitz, Rüdiger J., Raymond F. Paloutzian, and Hans-Ferdinand Angel. "Processes of believing: Where do they come from? What are they good for?". *F1000Res* 5 (2016): 2573.

Sfez, Lucien. *L'utopie de la santé parfaite*. Colloque de Cerisy. Paris: Presses universitaires de France, 2001.

Sheldrake, Philip F. *Explorations in Spirituality. History, Theology, dans Social Practice*. New York/Mahwah, NJ: Paulist Press, 2010.

Shorey, Ryan C., Michael J. Gawrysiak, Scott Anderson, and Gregory L. Stuart. "Dispositional mindfulness, spirituality, and substance use in predicting depressive symptoms in a treatment-seeking sample." *J Clin Psychol* 71, no. 4 (Apr 2015): 334–45.

Shuman, Joel J., and Keith G. Meador. *Heal Thyself. Spirituality, Medicine, and the Distorsion of Christianity*. Oxford: Oxford University Press, 2003.

Siddall, Philip J., Melanie Lovell, and Rod MacLeod. "Spirituality: What is Its Role in Pain Medicine?". *Pain Medicine* 16, no. 1 (2015–01–01 00:00:00 2015): 51–60.

Sinding, Christiane. "Une utopie médicale." In *Une utopie médicale La Sagesse du corps par Ernest Starling*, edited by Christiance Sinding. La fabrique du corps humain, 11–47. Arles: Acte Sud/INSERM, 1989.

Sloan, Richard P. *Blind Faith. The Unholy Alliance of Religion and Medicine*. New York: St. Martin's Press, 2006.

Sloan, Richard P., and Emilia Bagiella. "Data without a prayer." *Archives of Internal Medicine* 160, no. 12 (Jun 26 2000): 1870; author reply 77–8.

Sloan, Richard P., and Emilia Bagiella. "Religion and health." *Health Psychology* 20, no. 3 (May 2001): 228–9.

Sloan, Richard P., and Emilia Bagiella. "Spirituality and medical practice: a look at the evidence." *American Family Physician* 63, no. 1 (Jan 01 2001): 33–4.

Sloan, Richard P., Emilia Bagiella, and Thomas Powell. "Religion, spirituality, and medicine." *Lancet* 353, no. 9153 (Feb 20 1999): 664–7.

Sloan, Richard P., Emilia Bagiella, Larry VandeCreek, Margot Hover, Carlo Casalone, Trudi Jinpu Hirsch, Yusuf Hasan, Ralph Kreger, and Peter Poulos. "Should physicians prescribe religious activities?". *New England Journal of Medicine* 342, no. 25 (Jun 22 2000): 1913–6.

Smith, Jackie. "We believe it is better not to explicitly highlight spirituality." *Nursing Standard* 29, no. 37 (May 13 2015): 33.

Song, Mi-K., and Laura C. Hanson. "Relationships between psychosocial-spiritual well-being and end-of-life preferences and values in African American dialysis patients." *Journal of Pain and Symptom Management* 38, no. 3 (2009): 372–80.

Sournia, Jean-Charles. *Histoire de la médecine*. Sciences humaines et sociales. Paris: La Découverte, 1997.

Spinale, Joann, Scott D. Cohen, Prashant Khetpal, Rolf A. Peterson, Brenna Clougherty, Christina M. Puchalski, Samir S. Patel, and Paul L. Kimmel. "Spirituality, social support, and survival in hemodialysis patients." *Clinical Journal of the American Society of Nephrology* 3, no. 6 (Nov 2008): 1620–7.

Stewart, Donna E., and Tracy Yuen. "A systematic review of resilience in the physically ill." *Psychosomatics* 52, no. 3 (May-Jun 2011): 199–209.

Stolz, Jörg, Judith Könemann, Mallory Schneuwly Purdie, Thomas Englberger, and Michael Krüggeler. *Religion et spiritualité à l'ère de l'ego: profils de l'institutionnel, de l'alternatif, du distancié et du séculier [Religion and spirituality in the era of the ego. Institutional, alternative, distancing and secular profiles].* Genève: Labor et Fides, 2015.

Sulmasy, Daniel P. *The Healer's Calling. A Spirituality for Physicians and Other Health Care Professionals.* Mahwah, N.J.: Paulist Press, 1997.

Sulmasy, Daniel P. *The Rebirth of the Clinic. An Introduction to Spirituality in Health Care.* Washington, D.C.: Georgetown University Press, 2007.

Sulmasy, Daniel P. "A biopsychosocial-spiritual model for the care of patients at the end of life." *Gerontologist* 42 Spec No 3 (Oct 2002): 24–33.

Swift, Chris. "Omitting spirituality from NMC code disadvantages our patients." *Nursing Standard* 29, no. 38 (May 20 2015): 32–3.

Tanquerey, Adolphe. *Précis de théologie ascétique et mystique.* 8e ed. Paris: Desclée, 1923.

Tanyi, Ruth A., and Joan S. Werner. "Adjustment, spirituality, and health in women on hemodialysis." *Clinical Nursing Research* 12, no. 3 (Aug 2003): 229–45.

Taylor, Carol, Carol Lillis, and Priscilla LeMone. *Fundamentals of nursing: the art & science of nursing care.* 4th ed. Philadelphia: Lippincott, 2001.

Taylor, Charles. *Sources of the Self. The Making of the Modern Identity.* Cambridge, Ma: Harvard University Press, 1989.

Titus, Craig Steven. "Vertus." In *Dictionnaire encyclopédique d'éthique chrétienne*, edited by Laurent Lemoine, Eric Gaziaux and Denis Müller, 2073–93. Paris: Cerf, 2013.

Tracy, David. *The analogical imagination: Christian theology and the culture of pluralism.* New York: Crossroad, 1981.

Tubiana, Maurice. *Histoire de la pensée médicale. Les chemins d'Esculape.* Champs. Paris: Flammarion, 1995.

Underwood, Lynn G., and Jeanne A. Teresi. "The daily spiritual experience scale: development, theoretical description, reliability, exploratory factor analysis, and preliminary construct validity using health-related data." *Ann Behav Med* 24, no. 1 (Winter 2002): 22–33.

Vaghefi, Mahsa, Ali M. Nasrabadi, Seyed M. Golpayegani, Mohammad-R. Mohammadi, and Shahriar Gharibzadeh. "Spirituality and brain waves." *J Med Eng Technol* 39, no. 2 (Feb 2015): 153–8.

van der Walt, Freda, and Jeremias J. de Klerk. "Workplace spirituality and job satisfaction." *Int Rev Psychiatry* 26, no. 3 (Jun 2014): 379–89.

van Elk, Michiel, and André Aleman. "Brain mechanisms in religion and spirituality: An integrative predictive processing framework." *Neurosci Biobehav Rev* 73 (Feb 2017): 359–78.

Varambally, Shivarama, and Bengaluru N. Gangadhar. "Yoga: a spiritual practice with therapeutic value in psychiatry." *Asian J Psychiatr* 5, no. 2 (Jun 2012): 186–9.

Vésale, André. *La fabrique du corps humain.* La fabrique du corps humain. Edited by Claire Ambroselli. Arles: Actes Sud/INSERM, 1987[1543].

Vicini, Andrea. "La loi morale naturelle: perspectives internationales pour la réflexion bioéthique contemporaine." *Transversalités* 122 (2012): 125–51.

Vicini, Andrea. "Respecting life: theology and bioethics." *Journal of the Society of Christian Ethics* 35, no. 1 (2015 2015): 196–99.

Vieten, Cassandra, Shelley Scammell, Ron Pilato, Ingrid Ammondson, Kenneth I. Pargament, and David Lukoff. "Spiritual and religious competencies for psychologists." *Psychology of Religion and Spirituality* 5, no. 3 (2013): 129–44.

Vonarx, Nicolas. "De Bronislaw Malinowski à Virginia Henderson: révélation sur l'origine anthropologique d'un modèle de soins infirmiers." *Aporia* 2, no. 4 (2010): 19–28.

Vonarx, Nicolas, and Mireille Lavoie. "Soins infirmiers et spiritualité: d'une démarche systématique à l'accueil d'une expérience." *Revue internationale de soins palliatifs* 26, no. 4 (2011): 313–19.

Waaijman, Kees. *Spirituality: forms, foundations, methods.* Studies in spirituality Supplement. Vol. 8, Dudley, Mass: Peeters, 2002.

Wachholtz, Amy B., and Michelle J. Pearce. "Does spirituality as a coping mechanism help or hinder coping with chronic pain?". *Current Pain and Headache Reports* 13, no. 2 (Apr 2009): 127–32.

Walton-Moss, Benita, Ellen M. Ray, and Kathleen Woodruff. "Relationship of spirituality or religion to recovery from substance abuse: a systematic review." *J Addict Nurs* 24, no. 4 (Oct-Dec 2013): 217–26; quiz 27–8.

Walton, Joni. "Finding a balance: a grounded theory study of spirituality in hemodialysis patients." *Nephrology Nursing Journal* 29, no. 5 (Oct 2002): 447–56; discussion 57.

Weber, Max. *L'éthique protestante et l'esprit du capitalisme.* Paris: Plon, 1964.

Weinstein, Faye, Aryeh Bernstein, Talya Kapenstein, Elana Penn, and Steven H. Richeimer. "Spirituality Assessments and Interventions in Pain Medicine." Vertical Health LLC, http://www.practicalpainmanagement.com/treatments/psychological/spirituality-assessments-interventions-pain-medicine.

Wexler, Isaiah D., and Benjamin W. Corn. "An existential approach to oncology: meeting the needs of our patients." *Current Opinion in Supportive & Palliative Care* 6, no. 2 (2012): 275–79.

White, Kevin. "Parsons, American Sociology of Medicine and the Sick Role." In *An Introduction to the Sociology of Health and Illness*, 105–18. Los Angeles, Ca.: Sage, 2009.

WHO. "Preamble to the Constitution of the World Health Organization." https://www.who.int/about/fr/.

WHO. *La Charte de Bangkok pour la promotion de la santé à l'heure de la mondialisation.* 2005. http://www.who.int/healthpromotion/conferences/6gchp/BCHP_fr.pdf.

Wildes, Kevin W. "Religion in bioethics: a rebirth." *Christ Bioeth* 8, no. 2 (Aug 2002): 163–74.

Wright, Andrew. *Spirituality and education.* London: Falmer Press, 2000.

Yong, Jinsun, Juhu Kim, Junyang Park, Imsun Seo, and John Swinton. "Effects of a spirituality training program on the spiritual and psychosocial well-being of hospital middle manager nurses in Korea." *J Contin Educ Nurs* 42, no. 6 (Jun 2011): 280–8.

Yumba, François. *Les patients perdus de vue dans la prise en charge du Sida. Articulation entre santé, spiritualité et salut à partir de leur vécu à Kinshasa.* Théologies pratiques. Edited by Gilles Routhier. Bruxelles: Lumen vitae, 2017.

Zinnbauer, Brian J., Kenneth I. Pargament, Allie B. Scott. "The Emerging Meanings of Religiousness and Spirituality: Problems and Prospects." *Journal of Personality* 67, no. 6 (1999): 889–919.

Zoloth, Laurie. "Religion and the public discourse of bioethics." *Med Ethics* (Burlingt Mass) (Fall 1999): 1–2. *Dictionnaire de la vie spirituelle.* Paris: Cerf, 1983.

Zuckerman, Phil. *Faith no more: why people reject religion.* New York: Oxford University Press, 2012.

Index nominum

https://doi.org/10.1515/9783110638950-014

Index rerum

https://doi.org/10.1515/9783110638950-015